E. Fleck, E. Frantz (Eds.)

Complications in PTCA

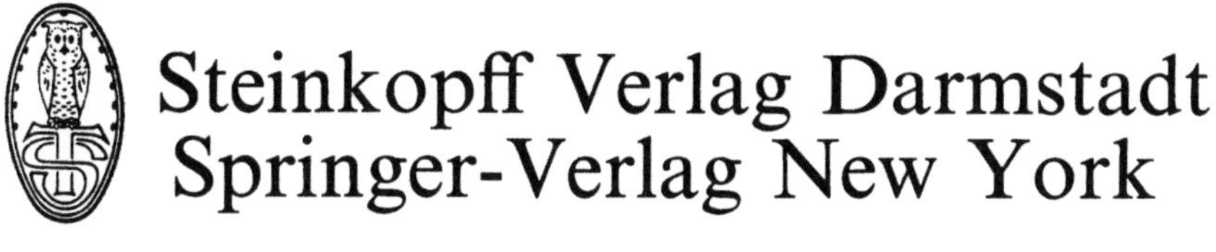

Steinkopff Verlag Darmstadt
Springer-Verlag New York

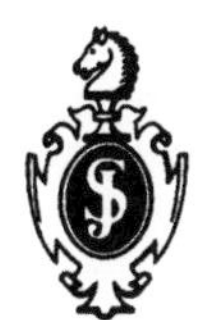

The Editors:
Prof. Dr. med. Eckart Fleck
Dr. med. Eckart Frantz
Klinik für Innere Medizin – Kardiologie
Deutsches Herzzentrum Berlin
Augustenburger Platz 1
1000 Berlin 65, FRG

CIP-Titelaufnahme der Deutschen Bibliothek
Complications in PTCA / E. Fleck ; E. Frantz (ed.). –
Darmstadt : Steinkopff ; New York : Springer, 1990
  ISBN-13:978-3-642-85396-8   e-ISBN-13:978-3-642-85394-4
  DOI: 10.1007/978-3-642-85394-4
NE: Fleck, Eckart [Hrsg.]

Medical Editorial: Sabine Müller – English Editor: James C. Willis – Production: Heinz J. Schäfer

Type-setting: The Alden Press, London

Printed on acid-free paper

Preface

Percutaneous Transluminal Coronary Angioplasty is presently the widest used non-surgical method for the treatment of stenotic lesions in coronary artery disease. Continuous development of the procedure and equipment has made complex and multi-vessel-interventions possible and has led to other techniques of intravascular angioplasty.

In reviewing current results, this volume pays particular attention to causes, incidence, circumstances, recognition, treatment and outcome of complications of PTCA; it also considers restenosis, which still occurs at an unsatisfactory high rate after primarily successful procedures.

To deal with these topics, experts on PTCA met to discuss their experiences and insights into peculiar aspects of complications in PTCA. The discussion was subdivided into:

Recognition of complications;
Complications in new interventional techniques;
Management of complications; and
Restenosis after angioplasty.

The question of whether angiographic and pathological characteristics of sclerotic lesions allow the identification of complication-prone lesions in advance is discussed in the first chapter. One paper deals with the state of the art of digital cardiac imaging, which enables the operator to have an early knowledge of and adequate reaction to possible complications occurring during angioplasty. Special attention is directed to the so-called "high-risk"-PTCA, detailing the clinical variables, in order to have better knowledge about patients with a higher probability of unsuccessful or complicated procedures.

Coronary atherectomy, angioscopy, stent implantation, and rotablation are new techniques that are covered in the second chapter. An investigation of special equipment for recanalization of chronic total occlusions is reported, and a review of actual reports on complications in conventional and new techniques is included.

Management of complications includes immediate re-dilatation, use of perfusion catheter and stent implantation, as well as emergency surgical interventions. Techniques, equipment, handling, and outcome figures are discussed in the third chapter.

The "restenosis"-chapter deals with angiographical and clinical characteristics of patients and vessel lesions, in which restenosis is most often observed. Pathological findings are reported to facilitate the understanding of possible pathogenetic factors of this still too frequent complication after PTCA.

Instead of conclusions, the final remarks consist of recommendations: Geoffrey A. Hartzler gives advice for adequate patient selection and angioplasters' training in order to prevent PTCA complications. The intention of this entire volume should be most evident: to aid in the prevention and management of complications after coronary angioplasty.

E. Fleck

Contents

The Authors

Dr. Frits W.H.M. Bär
Department of Cardiology
Academic Hospital of Maastricht
P.O. Box 1918
NL-6201 BX Maastricht
The Netherlands

Dr. Kevin J. Beatt MB BS MRCP
Departement of Cardiovascular Medicine
Charing Cross and Westminster Medical
  School
Horseferry Road
London SW1P 2AP
United Kingdom

Dr. A. Buchwald
Abteilung für Kardiologie, Universitäts-
  klinik
Robert-Koch-Straße 40
3400 Göttingen
FRG

Dr. C. Düber
Institut für Klinische Strahlenkunde Univer-
  sitätskliniken
Johannes-Gutenberg-Universität
Langenbeckstraße 1
6500 Mainz
FRG

Prof. Dr. Raimund Erbel FACC FESC
II. Medizinische Klinik Universitätskliniken
Johannes-Gutenberg-Universität
Langenbeckstraße 1
6500 Mainz
FRG

Prof. Dr. Eckart Fleck
Klinik für Innere Medizin – Kardiologie
Deutsches Herzzentrum Berlin
Augustenburger Platz 1
1000 Berlin 65,
FRG

Dr. Eckart Frantz
Klinik für Innere Medizin – Kardiologie
Deutsches Herzzentrum Berlin
Augustenburger Platz 1
1000 Berlin 65
FRG

PD Dr. Christian W. Hamm
II. Medizinische Klinik
Abteilung für Kardiologie
Universitätskrankenhaus Eppendorf
Martinistraße 52
2000 Hamburg 55
FRG

Geoffrey O. Hartzler M.D.
Cardiovascular Consultants, Inc.
4320 Wornall Road, Suite 20-II
Kansas City, MO 64111
USA

Dr. Martin Höher
Abteilung für Kardiologie-Pneumologie-
  Angiologie, Universität Ulm
Robert-Koch-Straße 8
7900 Ulm
FRG

Dr. Jürgen Krülls-Münch
Klinik für Innere Medizin – Kardiologie
Deutsches Herzzentrum Berlin
Augustenburger Platz 1
1000 Berlin 65
FRG

Dr. Audrey v. Pölnitz
Klinikum Großhadern
Medizinische Klinik I
Marchioninistraße 15
8000 München 70
FRG

Dr. Hans J. Rupprecht
II. Medizinische Klinik
Universitätskliniken
Johannes-Gutenberg-Universität
Langenbeckstraße 1
6500 Mainz
FRG

PD Dr. Wolfgang Rutsch
Medizinische Klinik und Poliklinik,
  Abteilung
Innere Medizin mit Schwerpunkt
  Kardiologie und
Pulmologie, Universitätsklinikum Rudolf
  Virchow
Freie Universität Berlin
Spandauer Damm 130
1000 Berlin 19
FRG

Dr. Dieter Vaterrodt
Klinik für Herz- und Kreislauferkrankungen
Deutsches Herzzentrum München
Lothstraße 11
8000 München 2
FRG

Dr. Henning Warnecke
Klinik für Herz-, Thorax- und
  Gefäßchirurgie
Deutsches Herzzentrum Berlin
Augustenburger Platz 1
1000 Berlin 65
FRG

Recognition of Complications

Lesion Types Correlating with High Incidence of Complications after PTCA

D. Vaterrodt, S. Dacian, J. Dirschinger, W. Rudolph

German Heart Center, Munich, FRG

Introduction

The rate of major complications during peructaneous transluminal coronary angiography (PTCA) remained unchanged or declined during the last decade with growing operator experience and ongoing improvements in balloon and wire technology, despite the fact that today's patient population might be expected to have a significantly higher risk for complications because of substantial differences in baseline characteristics such as multi-vessel disease, poor left ventricular function, and increased age. This fact has been clearly demonstrated by comparison of complication rates in the initial NHLBI PTCA registry cohort of 1977–1981, and the recent 1985/86 cohort [5,6,7,11].

In the vast majority the cause of a major complication was the acute occlusion of the vessel after an initially successful dilatation, typically with an extensive dissection or intimal tear. Spasm or thrombosis were rarely the principal mechanism, despite the fact that dissection and thrombosis may be very difficult to distinguish angiographically [23].

This study was undertaken to determine the incidence of acute occlusion and to identify lesion types associated with acute occlusion by definition of morphological characteristics in angiograms obtained prior to or during PTCA in a current patient population with expanded indications for the procedure, compared to the initial years, with high operator experience and after introduction of ultra low-profile balloon catheters.

Methods

Patient population

The study was started in April 1988. Up to May 1989, 650 elective PTCA procedures (from a total of 1000 procedures planned to be included) were performed in our institute. Excluded were PTCA attempts in the setting of an acute myocardial infarction. With an average of 1.9 attempted lesions per patient, 1235 lesions form the basis for this prelimary analysis. Multi-vessel disease was present in 54% of all cases, status post coronary artery bypass grafting in 4%. One-third of the patients had an impaired left ventricular function, 9% with an ejection fraction of less than 40%. The mean age was 57 years; 11% were females.

PTCA procedure

PTCA was performed with a femoral approach by use of 8F guiding catheters. Ultra low-profile balloon catheters with an outer deflated balloon diameter between 0.5 and 0.9 mm were chosen in order to have an inflated balloon diameter that approximated or slightly exceeded the pre- and poststenotic normal luminal diameter of the vessel. In case of large dissections post PTCA the patient was monitored in the cath lab for 15 to 30 min, mostly with the guiding catheter still across the lesion in order to be able to redilate immediately in case of acute occlusion. After PTCA patients were taken to a post-procedural ward where they were monitored until sheath removal the day after PTCA. Clinicas status, ECG, CK levels, and the PTT were obtained immediately after PTCA and at 4, 8, and 12 h.

The medical regimen pre, during, and post PTCA included an extensive antithrombotic and antispastic treatment with ASA 350 mg once daily, started at least 1 day before the procedure in 96% of all patients, and a dextrane infusion of 500 ml at 6 h prior to PTCA for a maximal anti-platelet effect. Heparin was administered in a dose of 10 000 to 15 000 units via a groin puncture. Further, 5 000 units were repeated hourly during the procedure. Nitrates and calcium channel blockers were given orally. Additionally, during the procedure nitrates and/or calcium channel blockers were administered intracoronarily or sublingually when spasm occurred. After PTCA all patients were kept on heparin for 24 h to achieve a two- to three-fold increase in partial thromboplasin time (PTT). Nitrates and calcium channel blockers were continued also for 1 day, and ASA was continued for 6 months.

Acute occlusion

Acute occlusion was defined as angiographic evidence of complete occlusion and/or clinical or ECG evidence of myocardial ischemia related to a dilated vessel, leading either to redilation, emergency coronary artery bypass grafting or myocardial infarction during or after an initially successful PTCA, up until hospital discharge.

Data collection

Data was recorded prospectively by a physician and entered into a computerized data bank. The following angiographic criteria was used:
  - location in the native coronary artieries by bypass grafts;
  - calcification of the stenosis, detected by fluoroscopy appearance;
  - curve with an angulation of more than 45° within the dilated segment;
  - diffuse disease with at least three 50% narrowings in the vessel or luminal irregularities present in one-third of the vessel;
  - eccentric lesions of type I or type II, according to the definition of Ambrose [1] with smooth borders and a broad neck or irregular borders or a narrow neck, respectively;
  - ostial stenosis;
  - side branch originating from the stenosis; and
  - side branch originating beside the stenosis, but within the dilated segment;
  - stenosis of 90% or more diameter reduction;
  - preexisting thrombus;
  - ulceration/aneurysma; and
  - as parameters available during the procedure: dissection or intimal tear: grade 0 = no angiographic evidence; grade 1 = slight linear intraluminal filling defect without contrast staining; grade 2 = slight filling defect with contrast staining; grade 3 = intraluminal filling defect at full balloon length and contrast staining or widening at the site of dilatation with extraluminal contrast staining; and
  - thrombus formation during the procedure.

Statistical analysis

Statistical analysis was performed with the chi-square significance test to assess differences in categorical variables. Significane was defined as a probability value (p) of less than 0.05.

4

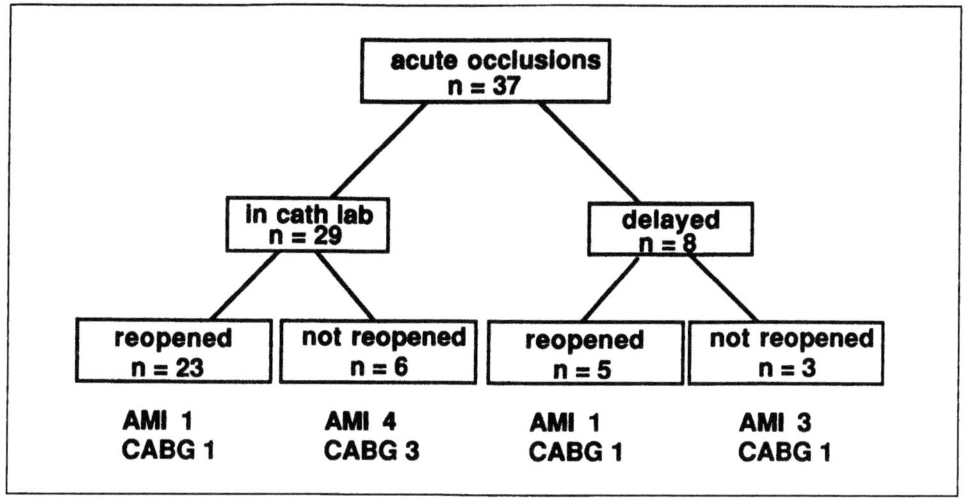

Fig. 1. Management and outcome of acute occlusions.

Results

Primary success rate, defined as residual stenosis of maximal 50% diameter reduction, was 95%. Acute occlusion occurred in 37 cases (in 5.7% of all patients or in 3% of all lesions attempted). Overall major complication rate was 2.9% with myocardial infarction in 1.7%, emergency coronary artery bypass grafting in 0.9% and death in 0.3%. Seventy-eight percent of all occlusions developed while the patient was still in the cath lab, most with the wire still across the lesion. In only eight patients did occlusion occur later, in a range of from 10 min to 76 h.

Twenty-eight of the 37 acute occlusions (76%) could be reopened by immediate redilation. Figure 1 shows the management and outcome of these cases.

The analysis of angiographic characteristics shows no significant difference in risk of occlusion between sites of lesions in the native coronary arteries or bypass grafts. There was a trend toward a higher pcercentage of patients with multi-vessel disease in the occlusion group which did not reach statistical significance (Table 1).

Lesion characteristics correlating significantly with acute occlusion were ostial involvement with 19% in the occlusion group vs. 9.6% in uncomplicated cases, stenoses in a curve of more than 45° (49% vs. 23%), lesions with a side branch originating from the stenosis (43% vs. 20%), eccentric stenoses type II (46% vs. 26%), stenoses longer than 6 mm (58% vs. 39%), diffuse diseased vessel (39% vs. 14%), and high-grade stenoses of 90% diameter reduction or more with 54% in the occlusion group vs. 30% in uncomplicated cases (Table 2).

No correlation could be found for lesion calcification, stenosis length less than 6 mm, eccentric lesions type I, lesions with side branches originating from the segment affected by the balloon but not from the stenosis itself, preexisting thrombus, ulceration/aneurysma, and thrombus formation during the procedure. The analysis of the angiographic extent of dissection during or immediately after the procedure showed that no lesion of the occlusion group was immediately post PTCA without signs of dissection, compared to 38% in the control group. A slight or moderate dissection was present in one-third of complicated cases vs. half of the control cases and a severe dissection could be detected in 68% in the occlusion group, but only in 12% of uncomplicated cases (Table 3). Table 4 shows that the calculated absolute risks to develop acute occlusion in presence of the

Table 1. Location of stenosis and incidence of acute occlusions.

	% occlusion group n = 37	% non occlusion group n = 1198	p value
- LM	0	0.2	n.s.
- LAD prox.	37.9	34.2	n.s.
- med.	16.2	10.8	n.s.
- dist.	2.7	2.6	n.s.
- other	2.7	2.4	n.s.
- LCX prox.	5.4	8.2	n.s.
- dist.	2.7	6.7	n.s.
- other	2.7	7.1	n.s.
-RCA prox.	10.8	9.9	n.s.
- med.	13.5	9.3	n.s.
- dist.	2.7	3.6	n.s.
- other	0	1	n.s.
- ACVB prox. anast.	0	1.5	n.s.
- body	2.7	2	n.s.
- dist. anast.	0	0.5	n.s.
- IMA	0	0	n.s.
-MVD	65	54	n.s.

defined morphologic characteristics amounts to 4.3–7.7%, compared with the 3% average risk per lesion of the entire group. Again, the most powerful predictor was the extent of dissection immediately post PTCA. Cases with severe dissection, as defined previosuly, evolved acute occlusion in 16% compared to 1.9% if dissection appeared angiographically, either as slight or moderate.

Table 2. Morphologic characteristics and incidence of acute occlusions.

	% occlusion group n = 37	% non occl. group n = 1198	p value
— ostial stenosis	19	9.6	< 0.05
— curve > 45 degrees	49	23	< 0.05
— side branch from stenosis	43	20	< 0.05
— eccentric stenosis type II	46	26	< 0.05
— stenosis length $\geq$ 6 mm	59	39	< 0.05
— diffuse disease	39	14	< 0.05
— stenosis $\geq$ 90% diam. reduct.	54	30	< 0.05
— calcification (any degree)	29	21	n.s.
— stenosis length < 6 mm	41	61	n.s.
— eccentric stenosis type I	30	29	n.s.
— side branch in dilat. segm.	38	31	n.s.
— preexisting thrombus	8	5	n.s.
— ulceration/aneurysma	3	2	n.s.
— thrombus formation	3	1	n.s.
— dissection severe	68	12	< 0.05

Table 3. Angiographic appearance of dissection post PTCA in complicated and uncomplicated cases.

	% occlusion group n = 37	% non occlusion group n = 1198	p value
No dissection	0	38	< 0.05
slight/moderate	32	50	n.s.
severe	68	12	< 0.05

Discussion

The analysis of the first 650 PTCA procedures included in this study shows that the incidence of acute occlusion during or after PTCA until hospital discharge averages up to 3% per attempted lesion or 5.7% per patient in a current patient population. In only 1.2% of all cases, the occlusion occurred after the patient had left the cath lab.

The analysis of morphological factors in angiograms obtained prior to or during PTCA identified seven lesion characteristics associated significantly with acute occlusion: ostial involvement, stenosis in a curve, lesions with a side branch originating from the stenosis itself, eccentric stenoses type II with irregular borders or a narrow neck, as defined by Ambrose [1], stenosis length of more than 6 mm, diffuse disease, and high-grade stenoses of 90% diameter reduction or more.

In our study the site of the lesion in the native coronary arteries or coronary artery bypass grafts showed no correlation with acute occlusion, as published by Ellis and coworkers and Bredlau for the Emory experience [3,8]. However, the initial NHLBI registry reported a higher percentage of right coronary artery stenoses in cases complicated by acute occlusion [7]. Topol found a significantly higher occlusion rate of 9.4% leading to emergency coronary artery bypass grafting in ostial RCA stenoses [22]. Ostial involvement was also a risk factor in our study.

Platko defined aortocoronary vein grafts older than 36 months as a risk group [17]. Because of the small proportion of graft stenoses in our own patients it is not possible to identify this risk group in the present study.

Eccentric stenoses are uniformly considered to be at higher risk [3,4,8,15,19]. In our experience with a high proportion of eccentric stenoses, it was mainly the eccentric stenosis type II, as defined by Ambrose [1], which led to acute closure. Similar to the nondiscrete lesions in the NHLBI registry, diffusely diseased vessels in the Emory analysis and also in our own study were found to be risk factors as well as was the long lesion with a length of at least 6–10 mm or 2 luminal diameters [4,7,8,15,18].

There is evidence that high-grade stenosis with a diameter reduction of 90% or more leads to a significantly increased occlusion rate [4,7]. The Emory group, however, comes to another conclusion, but one has to consider that the high-grade stenoses in their series amounted to only 9% compared to 37–52% in others, including in our study [8].

Lesions in a curve or with a side branch originating from the stenosis itself, as shown by Ellis from the Emory group, were in our study also at a higher risk [8,16].

A correlation between any degree of lesion calcification and closure could not be found in the majority of studies [3,8].

It cannot be excluded that thrombus may play a significant role in this field, but its importance is very difficult to be assessed by angiography [2,8,10,13,14,20,21]. In our own experience with an extensive antithrombotic medication pre, during, and after PTCA, thrombus formation appeared angiographically in only four of 1235 treated vessels. Other diagnostic methods such as angioscopy may be required to assess the incidence of thrombus formation during the procedure.

Table 4. Risk of acute occlusions in the presence of morphological risk factors.

	occlusion rate per vessel (%)
total	3
ostial stenosis	5.7
curve > 45 degrees	6.1
side branch from stenosis	6.3
eccentric lesion type II	5.2
stenosis length ≥ 6 mm	4.3
diffuse disease	7.7
stenosis ≥ 90% diam. reduct.	5
dissection severe	16

Uniformly, the presence of a dissection or intimal tear after PTCA is considered to be highly predictive of acute closure [3,8,9,10,12,19,20]. According to our own data, only the severe dissection with a length larger than the dilated segment and contrast staining or widening of the dilated segment with extra-luminal contrast showed a highly significant correlation, whereas the slight or moderate dissection was not associated with acute occlusion.

The presence of multiple angiographic risk factors will probably lead to a further increase of the complication rate [8]. At the present time the number of 650 patients included in this ongoing study is still too small to demonstrate this fact with statistical significance.

In conclusion, the identification of angiographic risk factors available pre PTCA associated with a higher complication rate may be helpful in patient selection and in defining the PTCA strategy. Another very important angiographic predictor of acute occlusion during or after PTCA is the presence of an extensive dissection, as defined above, and can be assessed during the procedure.

Conclusion

In order to determine the incidence of acute coronary occlusion during or after PTCA in a current patient population after introduction of ultra low-profile balloon catheters and to identify lesion types associated with high incidence of occlusions, 650 consecutive PTCA procedures were analyzed prospectively. The incidence amounted to 5.7% of all patients or 3.7% of all attempted lesions. Angiographic characteristics related to acute occlusion were ostial involvement, stenosis in a curve of more than 45°, lesions with a side branch originating from the stenosis itself, eccentric stenoses with irregular borders on a narrow neck, stenosis length of more than 6 mm, diffuse disease, and high-grade stenoses with 90% diameter reduction or more. No correlation could be found for lesion calcification, stenosis length of less than 6 mm, eccentric stenoses with smooth borders and a broad neck, lesions with side branches originating from the dilated segment but not from the stenosis itself, preexisting thrombus/ulceration/aneurysma and the lesion's site. The most important predictor available during the procedure is severe dissection with a length larger than the dilated segment and contrast staining or widening of the dilated segment with extraluminal contrast staining, whereas the slight or moderate dissection were not associated with acute collusion.

References

1. Ambrose JA, Wintwers SL, Stern A, Eng A, Teichholz LE, Gorlin R, Fuster V (1985) Angiographic Morphololgy and the Pathogenesis of Unstable Angina Pectoris. JACC 5: 509–616

2. Barnathan ES, Schwartz JS, Taylor L, Laskey WK, Kleaveland JP, Kussmaul WG, Hirshfeld JW (1987) Aspirin and Dipyridamole in the Prevention of Acute Coronary Thrombosis Complicating Coronary Angioplasty. Circulation 76: 125–134.
3. Bredlau CE, Roubin GS, Leimgruber PP, Douglas JS, King SB, Gruentzig AR (1985) In-hospital Morbidity and Mortality in Patients undergoing Elective Coronary Angioplasty. Circulation 72: 1044–1052.
4. Cowley MJ, Dorros G, Kelsey SF, Van Raden M, Detre KM (1984) Acute Coronary Events Associated with Percutaneous Transluminal Coronary Angioplasty. Am J Cardiol 53: 12C–16C
5. Detre K, Holubkov R, Kelsey S, Cowley M, Kent K, Williams D, Myler R, Faxon D, Holmes D, Bourassa M, Block P, Gosselin A, Bentivoglio L, Leatherman L, Dorros G, King S, Galichia J, Al-Bassam M, Leon M, Robertson T, Passamani E (1988) Percutaneous Transluminal Coronary Angioplasty in 1985–1986 and 1977–1981. The National Heart, Lung, and Blood Institute Registry. N Engl J Med 318: 265–270
6. Dorros G, Cowley MJ, Janke L, Kelsey SF, Mullin SM, Van Raden M (1984) In-Hospital Mortality Rate in the National Heart, Lung, and Blood Institute Percutaneous Transluminal Coronary Angioplasty Registry. Am J Cardiol 53: 17C–21C
7. Dorros G, Cowley MJ, Simpson J, Bentivoglio LG, Block PC, Bourassa M, Detre K, Gosselin AJ, Grüntzig AR, Kelsey SF, Kent KM, Mock MB, Mullin SM, Myler RK, Passamani ER, Stertzer SH, Williams DO (1983) Percutaneous Transluminal Coronary Angioplasty: Report of Complications from the National Heart, Lung, and Blood Instituten PTCA Registry. Circulation 67: 723–730
8. Ellis SG, Roubin GS, King SB, Douglas JS, Weintraub WS, Thomas RG, Cox WR (1988) Angiographic and Clinical Predictors of Acute Closure After Native Vessel Coronary Angioplasty. Circulation 77: 372–379
9. Gaul G, Hollman J, Simpfendorfer C, Franco I (1989) Acute Occlusion in Multiple Lesion Coronary Angioplasty: Frequency and Management. JACC 13: 283–288
10. Hollman J, Gruentzig AR, Douglas JS, King SB, Ischinger T, Meier B (1983) Acuta Occlusion after Percutaneous Transluminal Coronary Angioplasty – a New Approach. Circulation 68: 725–732
11. Holmes DR, Holubkov R, Vliestra RE, Kelsey SF, Reeder GS, Dorros G, Williams DO, Cowley MJ, Faxon DP, Kent KM, Bentivoglio LG, Detre K (1988) Comparison of Complications During Percutaneous Transluminal Coronary Angioplasty From 1977 to 1981 and From 1985 to 1986: The National Heart, Lung, and Blood Institute Percutaneous Transluminal Coronary Angioplasty Registry. JACC 12: 1149–55
12. Ischinger T, Gruentzig AR, Meier B, Galan K (1986) Coronary Dissection and total Coronary Occlusion Associated with Percutaneous Transluminal Coronary Angioplasty: Significance of Initial Angiographic Morphology of Coronary Stenoses. Circulation 74: 1371–1378
13. Mabin TA, Holmes DA, Smith HC, Vliestra RE, Bove AA, Reeder GS, Chesebro JH, Bresnahan JF, Orzulak TA (1985) Intracoronary Thrombus: Role in Coronary Occlusion Complicating Percutaneous Transluminal Coronary Angioplasty. JACC 5: 192–202
14. Marquis JF, Schwartz L, Aldridge H, Majid P, Henderson M, Matushinsky E (1984) Acute Coronary Artery Occlusion During Percutaneous Transluminal Coronary Angioplasty Treated by Redilation of the Occluded Segment. JACC 4: 1268–71
15. Meier B, Gruentzig AR, Hollman J, Ischinger T, Bradford JM (1983) Does Length or Eccentricity of Coronary Stenoses Influence the Outcome of Transluminal Dilation? Circulation 67: 497–499
16. Meier B, Gruentzig AR, King SB, Douglas JS, Hollman J, Ischinger T, Aueron F, Galan K (1984) Risk of Side Branch Occlusion During Coronary Angioplasty. Am J Cardiol 53: 10–14
17. Platko WP, Hollman J (1988) Vein Graft Angioplasty (PTCA): Immediate and Long Term Results. Circulation 78 (suppl. 2): 376
18. Roubin GS, Lin S, Niederman A, Weintraub WS, Douglas JS, King SB (1987) Clinical and Anatomic Descriptors for a Major Complication Following PTCA. JACC 9: 20A
19. Simpfendorfer C, Belardi J, Bellamy G, Galan K, Franco I, Hollman J (1987) Frequency, Management and Follow-up of Patients with Acute Coronary Occlusions After Percutaneous Transluminal Coronary Angioplasty. Am J Cardiol 59: 267–269
20. Sinclair IN, McCrabe CH, Sipperly ME, Baim DS (1988) Predictors, Therapeutic Options and Long Term Outcome of Abrupt Reclosure. Am J Cardiol 61: 61G–66G
21. Sugrue DD, Holmes DR, Smith HC, Reeder GS, Lane GE, Vliestra RE, Bresnahan JF, Hammes LN, Piehler JM (1986). Br Heart J 56: 62–66
22. Topol EJ, Ellis S, Fisherman-Rosen J, Leimgruber P, Myler RK, Stertzer SH, O'Neill WW, Roubin GS, Douglas JS, King SB (1987) Multicenter Study of Percutaneous Transluminal Angioplasty for Right Coronary Artery Ostial Stenosis. JACC 9: 20A

23. Topol EJ (1989) Emerging Strategies for Failed Percutaneous Transluminal Coronary Angioplasty. Am J Cardiol 63: 249–250

Author's address:
Dr. D. Vaterrodt
Deutsches Herzzentrum München
Klinik für Herz- und Kreislauferkrankungen
Lothstraße 11
8000 München 2, FRG

Pathologist's Findings after PTCA (The Mechanism of Angioplasty)

C. Düber

Institut für Klinische Strahlenkunde, Universitätskliniken, Mainz, FRG

Knowledge of the pathological changes induced by percutaneous transluminal coronary angioplasty (PTCA) is necessary to understand its complications.

The following discussion on the mechanisms of PTCA is based on own autopsy studies in six patients, who died after combined thrombolysis and PTCA for acute myocardial infarction and in another patient who died after elective PTCA [18, 27], and other autopsy studies reported in the literature [1, 3, 6, 13–15, 19–22, 25, 26, 29–37, 39–44, 46, 47].

At least six potential mechanisms of angioplasty have been discussed (Table 1). They are reviewed in the following.

Table 1. Potential mechanisms of angioplasty.

compression
redistribution
fluid extrusion
embolization
removal
wall injury and stretching

Compression

Compression or compaction of the atheromatous plaque was said to be the mechanism of angioplasty according to Dotter and Grüntzig in their early papers on PTA [16, 17, 23, 24].

In 1968, Dotter et al. [17] stated: "As a result of forceful dilatation with a catheter the lumen but not the artery is enlarged by compaction. . . . In effect transluminal dilatation by compression-remodelling converts an initally obstructing, thickened arterial core into a stable, in situ, autogenous tube with minimal trauma and maximum preservation of intimal continuity."

However, experimental studies have shown noncompressibility of the normal arterial wall [8] and atheromatous intimal lesions are composed of substances which are physically not compressible under pressure forces applied during angioplasty. In vitro studies by Chin et al. [12] have shown that plaque compaction accounts for 1–1.5% of luminal area increase of excised cadaver arteries. There has been no convincing evidence from pathological studies supporting plaque compression as a mechanism of angioplasty, although "compaction of the inner layer of intimal plaques" has been described [30].

Redistribution

Redistribution of the intimal plaque into a less obstructing configuration by lengthening the lesion, considered theoretically by Castaneda-Zuniga et al. [9–11], has been demonstrated in vitro and angiographically [45].

Although redistribution of plaque components cannot be verified directly by autopsy investigations, longitudinal and circumferential intimal tears indicate shear forces, which may lead to rearrangement of the plaque in axial direction. However, contribution of redistribution to luminal increase is thought to not be important.

Fluid extrusion

Extrusion of liquid plaque substances during angioplasty has been demonstrated in vitro by Chin et al. [12] and Kaltenbach et al. [28]. Its relative contribution to the overall increase in luminal cross-sectional area was 6–12% [12].

The possible role of this mechanism cannot be analyzed in autopsy studies. However, it seems unlikely that fluid extrusion is a significant mechanism in sclerotic and calcified plaques.

Embolization

Embolization of small amounts of superficial endothelial cells and lipid debris was detected occasionally during dilatation of atherosclerotic animal arteries by Block et al. [7] and Sanborn et al. [38]. Embolization of large solid plaque components has been described as a complication in case reports after PTCA [2] and PTA of peripheral arteries [26, 45].

In our studies release of lipid substances into the arterial lumen was observed in three patients with splitting of the fibrous cap of mixed plaques. Detachment of the whole plaque or major parts of it was not seen, despite extensive intimal tearing and subintimal dissection.

It is concluded from these observations, other autopsy studies, and clinical experience that distal embolization is neither an important mechanism nor a frequent complication of angioplasty. However, it may occur during dilatation of complex intimal lesions containing large amounts of lipid debris.

Removal

Retraction of ruptured intimal flaps and partial dissolution of atheromatous material has been considered to be a possible healing mechanism after PTCA with enlargement of luminal cross-sectional area [4, 5]. There is no evidence from our autopsy studies and observations of others supporting this suggestion.

Wall injury and stretching

Arterial wall injury was the predominant finding in our and other's autopsy studies. Incomplete or complete rupture of the inner portion of the arterial wall (intima and media) seems to be an inevitable and necessary event during successful PTCA.

In our studies intimal tears ranging from small fissures in the inner portion of the intima to complete splitting extending to the internal elastic lamina were constant findings in all patients. The tears occurred within the plaque or at the junction of normal and diseased intima.

Their orientation was always longitudinal. On cross section the tears were either radial or, more frequently, circumferential along preexisting layers within the plaque.

Splitting of the fibrous cap of a mixed atheromatous lesion with release of lipid debris into the arterial lumen was noted in two patients.

Subintimal dissection with separation of the intima from the media along the internal elastic lamina was seen in four patients with complete splitting of the intima.

Complete rupture of the media was observed in four patients with overlying intimal rupture. However, medial tears were also seen without histological changes of the adjacent intima.

Complete rupture of intima and media was associated with extensive submedial dissection in two patients.

Stretching of the grossly intact media and adventitia, or adventitia alone (in cases with complete rupture of intima and media), which constitutes formation of an aneurysm, was indicated by small or large gaps between intimal flaps causing redundancy of the outer layers and focal or complete necrosis of the media.

Congestion of adventitial blood vessels and a slight inflammatory reaction was noted in all patients. Bleeding within the connective tissue around the dilated part of the artery was seen both macroscopically and histologically in two cases. In another case extensive adventitial bleeding had caused hemopericardium. Morphological changes induced by PTCA (including the healing process discussed in the chapter: Pathologist's view on restenosis) are summarized in Fig. 1.

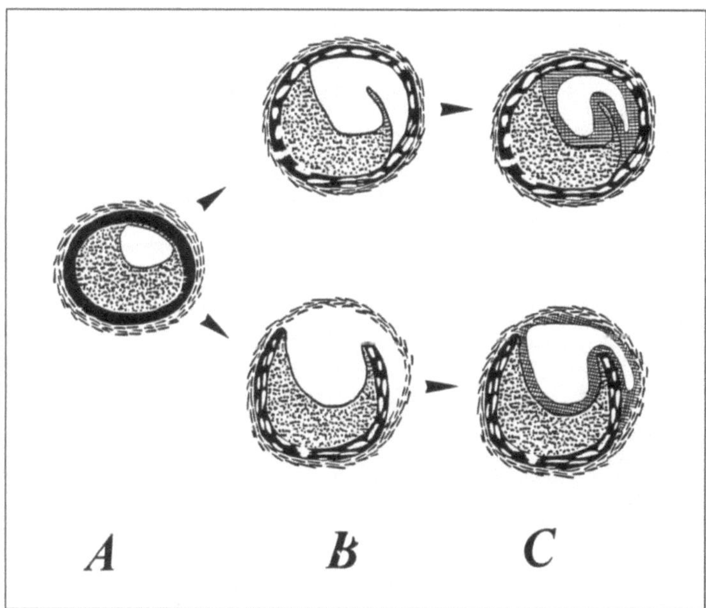

Fig. 1. Mechanisms of PTCA. A) Before PTCA. Stenosis by excentric intimal plaque; B) Early after PTCA: enlargement of luminal cross-sectional area induced by wall injury with rupture of intima and subintimal dissection (upper line) or intima and media with subintimal dissection (lower line) and stretching of media and adventitia (upper line) or adventia (lower line); C) Late after PTCA: neointima covering neoluminal surface and causing restenosis.

References

1. Adams CWM, Reidy J (1987) Renal artery pathology after percutaneous transluminal angioplasty. Atherosclerosis 67: 153–157
2. Auron F, Grüntzig A (1984) Distal embolization of a coronary artery bypass atheroma during percutaneous transluminal angioplasty. Am J Cardiol 53: 953–954
3. Austin GE, Ratliff NB, Hollman J, Phillips DF (1985) Intimal proliferation of smooth muscle cells as an explanation for recurrent coronary artery stenosis after percutaneous transluminal coronary angioplasty. J Am Coll Cardiol 6: 369–375
4. Block PC, Baughman KL, Pasternak RC, Fallon, JT (1980) Transluminal angioplasty: correlation of morphologic and angiographic findings in an experimental model. Circulation 61: 778–785
5. Block PC, Fallon JT, Elmer D (1980) Experimental angioplasty: lessons from the laboratory. Am J Roentgenol 135: 907–912
6. Block PC, Myler RK, Sterzer S, Fallon JT (1981) Morphology after transluminal angioplasty in human beings. New Engl J Med 305: 382–385
7. Block PC, Elmer D, Fallon JT (1982) Release of atherosclerotic debris after transluminal angioplasty. Circulation 65: 950–952
8. Carew TE, Vaishnav RN, Patel DJ (1968) Compressibility of the arterial wall. Circ Res 23: 61–68
9. Castaneda-Zuniga WR, Formanek A, Tadavarthy M, Vlodar Z, Edwards JE, Zollikofer C, Amplatz K (1980) The mechanism of angioplasty. Radiology: 135: 565–571
10. Castaneda-Zuniga WR, Amplatz K, Laerum F, Formanek A, Sibley R, Edwards J, Vlodaver Z (1981) Mechanics of angioplasty: an experimental approach. Radiographics 1: 1–14
11. Castaneda-Zuniga WR, Sibley R, Amplatz K (1984) The pathologic basis of angioplasty. Angiology 35: 195–205
12. Chin AK, Kinney TB, Rurik GW, Shoor PM, Fogarty TJ (1984) A physical measurement of the mechanics of transluminal angioplasty. Surgery 95: 196–200
13. Clouse ME, Tomashefski JF, Reinhold RE, Costello P (1981) Mechanical effect of balloon angioplasty: case report with histology. Am J Roentgenol 137: 869–871
14. Colavita PG, Ideker RE, Reimer KA, Hackel DB, Stack RS (1986) The spectrum of pathology associated with percutaneous transluminal coronary angioplasty during acute myocardial infarction. J Am Coll Cardiol 8: 855–860
15. de Morais CF, Lopes EA, Checchi H, Arie S, Pileggi F (1986) Percutaneous transluminal coronary angioplasty-histopathological analysis of nine necropsy cases. Virchow Arch A 410: 195–202
16. Dotter CT, Judkins MP (1964): Transluminal treatment of arteriosclerotic obstruction. Description of a new technique and a preliminary report of its application. Circulation 30: 654–670
17. Dotter CT, Rösch J, Judkins MP (1968) Transluminal dilatation of atherosclerotic stenosis. Surg Gyn Obst 127: 794–804
18. Düber C, Jungbluth A, Rumpelt HJ, Erbel R, Meyer J, Thoenes W (1986) Morphology of the coronary arteries after combined thrombolysis and percutaneous transluminal angioplasty for acute myocardial infarction. Am J Cardiol 58, 698–703
19. Essed CE, Van den Brand M, Becker AE (1983) Transluminal coronary angioplasty and early restenosis. Fibrocellular occlusion after wall laceration. Br Heart J 49: 393–396
20. Famularo M, Vasilomanolakis EC, Schrager B, Talbert W, Ellestad M (1983) Percutaneous transluminal angioplasty of aortocoronary saphenous vein graft. JAMA 249: 3347–3350
21. Fröhlich H, K100 C, Scheppokat KD (1984) Pathomorphologische Veränderungen nach perkutaner transluminaler Angioplastie. Fortschr Röntgenstr 140: 726–728
22. Giraldo AA, Esposo OM, Meis JM (1985) Intimal hyperplasia as a cause of restenosis after percutaneous transluminal coronary angioplasty. Arch Pathol Lab Med 109: 173–175
23. Grüntzig A (1978) Transluminal dilatation of coronary-artery stenosis. Lancet 1: 263
24. Grüntzig AR, Senning A, Siegenthaler WE (1979) Nonoperative dilatation of coronary-artery stenosis. Percutaneous transluminal coronary angioplasty. N Engl J Med 301: 61–68
25. Hoffman MA, Fallon JT, Greenfield AJ, Waltman AC, Athansoulis CA, Block CA (1981) Arterial pathology after percutaneous transluminal angioplasty. Am J Roentgenol 137: 147–149
26. Jester HG, Sinapius D (1978) Morphologic alterations after percutaneous transluminal recanalization of chronic femoral atherosclerosis. In: Zeitler E, Grüntzig A, Schoop W (editors): Percutaneous Vascular Recanalization. Berlin-Heidelberg-New York, Springer, pp 51–56
27. Jungbluth A, Düber C, Rumpelt HJ, Erbel R, Meyer J (1988) Koronararterienmorphologie nach perkutaner transluminaler Koronarangioplastie (PTCA) mit Hämoperikard. Z Kardiol 77: 125–129
28. Kaltenbach M, Beyer J, Klepzig H, Schmidts L, Hübner K (1982) Effects of 5 kg/cm² pressure on atherosclerotic vessel wall segments. In: Kaltenbach M, Grüntzig A, Rentrop K, Bussmann WD

(Editors): Transluminal Coronary Angioplasty and Intracoronary Thombolysis. Berlin-Heidelberg-New York, Springer, pp 189–193

29. Kohchi K, Takebayashi S, Block PC, Hiroki T, Nobuyoshi M (1987) Arterial changes after percutaneous transluminal coronary angioplasty. J Am Coll Cardiol 10: 592–599
30. Leu HJ (1983) The morphological concept of percutaneous transluminal angioplasty. In: Dotter CT, Grüntzig A, Schoop W, Zeitler E (editors): Percutaneous Transluminal Angioplasty. Berlin-Heidelberg-New York, Springer, pp 46–55
31. Mittal V, Karl EM, Atkinson JB, Virmani R (1986) Early and late morphologic changes after transluminal balloon angioplasty of the iliac arteries. Am J Cardiol 58: 182–184
32. Mizuno K, Kuritta A, Imazeki N (1984) Pathological findings after percutaneous transluminal coronary angioplasty. Br Heart J 52: 588–590
33. Mohacsy J, Bodrog I, Urai L (1984) Pathomorphology of the arterial wall following transluminal recanalization. Ann Radiol 27: 357–360
34. Myles JL, Zaidi A, Radliff NB, Tan TB, Hollman J (1988) Mechanisms of vessel injury during percutaneous transluminal angioplasty of saphenous vein bypass grafts and coronary arteries. Am J Cardiovasc Pathol 2: 133–136
35. Potkin BN, Roberts WC (1988) Effects of percutaneous transluminal coronary angioplasty on atherosclerotic plaques and relation of plaque composition and arterial size to outcome. Am J Cardiol 62: 41–50
36. Saber RS, Edwards WD, Holmes DR, Vlietstra RE, Reeder GS (1988) Balloon angioplasty of aorocoronary saphenous vein bypass grafts: a histopathologic study of six grafts from five patients with emphasis on restenosis and embolic complications. J Am Coll Cardiol 12: 1501–1509
37. Saffitz EJ, Rose TE, Oaks JB, Roberts WC (1983) Coronary artery rupture during coronary angioplasty. Am J Cardiol 51: 902–904
38. Sanborn TA, Faxon DP, Waugh, Small DM, Haudenschild C, Gottsman SB, Ryan TJ (1982) Transluminal angioplasty in experimental atherosclerosis. Analysis for embolization using an in vivo perfusion system. Circulation 66: 917–922
39. Schneider J, Grüntzig A (1985) Percutaneous transluminal angioplasty. Morphological findings in 3 patients. Path Res Prac 180: 348–352
40. Soward AL, Essed CE, Serruys PW (1985) Coronary arterial findings after accidental death immediately after successful percutaneous transluminal coronary angioplasty. Am J Cardiol 56: 794–795
41. Ueda M, Becker AE, Fujimoto T (1987) Pathological changes induced by repeated percutaneous transluminal coronary angioplasty. Br Heart J 58: 635–643
42. Waller BF, Gorfinkel HJ, Rogers FJ, Kent KM, Roberts WC (1984) Early and late morphological changes in major epicardial coronary arteries after percutaneous transluminal coronary angioplasty. Am J Cardiol 53: 42C–47C
43. Waller BF, Rothbaum DA, Pinkerton CA, Cowley MJ, Linnemeier TJ, Orr C, Irons M, Helmuth RA, Wills ER, Aust C (1987) Status of the myocardium and infarct-related coronary artery in 19 necropsy patients with acute recanalization using pharmacologic (streptokinase, r-tissue plasminogen activator), mechanical (percutaneous transluminal coronary angioplasty) or combined types of reperfusion therapy. Am J Coll Cardiol 9: 785–801
44. Waller BC, Pinkerton CA, Foster LN (1987) Morphologic evidence of accelerated left main coronary artery stenosis: a late complication of percutaneous transluminal balloon angioplasty of the proximal left anterior descending coronary artery. J Am Coll Cardiol 9: 1019–1023
45. Wolf GL, LeVeen RF, Ring EJ (1984) Potential mechanisms of angioplasty. Cardiovasc Intervent Radiol 7: 11–17
46. Wood WD (1982) Transluminal coronary angioplasty. N Engl J Med 306: 1055
47. Zarins CK, Lu C, Gewertz BL, Lyon RT, Rush DS, Glagov S (1982) Arterial disruption and remodelling following balloon dilatation. Surgery 92: 1086–1095

Author's address:
Dr C. Düber
Institut für Klinische Strahlenkunde
Universitätskliniken
Johannes-Gutenberg-Universität
Langenbeckstrasse 1
6500 Mainz, FRG

Digital Coronary Angiography: Relevance for Diagnosis and Invasive Treatment, Use of Quantitative Picture Interpretation, and Error Correction Modalities

E. Fleck and H. Oswald

German Heart Institute, Berlin, FRG

Summary

The application of new digital imaging systems in cardioangiography allows immediate diagnostic decisions in the cath lab based on quantitative parameters established during examination of the patient, thus supporting direct interventional treatments within the same setting. Easy digital image recording with optimized on-line image representation from digital storage by using algorithms for contour and contrast enhancement, and dynamic noise suppression is of high practical use and quality. The result is an image that is comparable or even superior to a conventional cine picture. These systems are available, not only for diagnostic purposes, but also for any type of intervention, and they are extremely helpful in case of complex anatomy or complications, because they use more direct decision supporting techniques.

Introduction

Digital angiography combined with image enhancement techniques, such as filtering, interframe gapfilling, single frame display, image post processing and quantitative image analysis has proven clinically useful. Especially for interventional procedures like PTCA, endartherectomy, etc., biplane x-ray systems additionally provide the user with pulsed flouroscopy to image details using x-ray doses that exceed conventional fluoroscopy. A high spatial (4.0 to 4.5 lp/mm), temporal ($< 150\,\mathrm{fr/s}$) and contrast resolution is the state of the art. The limitations of the conventional analog technique for adequate diagnostic interpretations are the insufficient contrast resolution for extreme projections or obese patients and – especially – those caused by delayed availability of the developed film. As long as diagnosis and subsequent acute intervention in the same setting was an uncommon situation in angiocardiographic labs, this disadvantage was not a real barrier. But now digital imaging and image processing allows a reasonable solution and handling. For this to be realized new digital methods had to generate images, as well as to process and display them, whereas digital subtraction techniques for coronary examination were insufficient.

These digital techniques provide images for on-line postprocessing and, by giving access to immediate diagnosis (even that based on quantifications) they are thus extremely helpful in interventions, and can be used as a starting point in improving traditional forms of diagnostic procedures and their order in the cath-lab. Quantitative analysis will certainly accelerate this development and enhance the technique.

Basic requirements for digital coronary angiographic systems

The following two distinctive features characterize a digital system for cardioangiography:

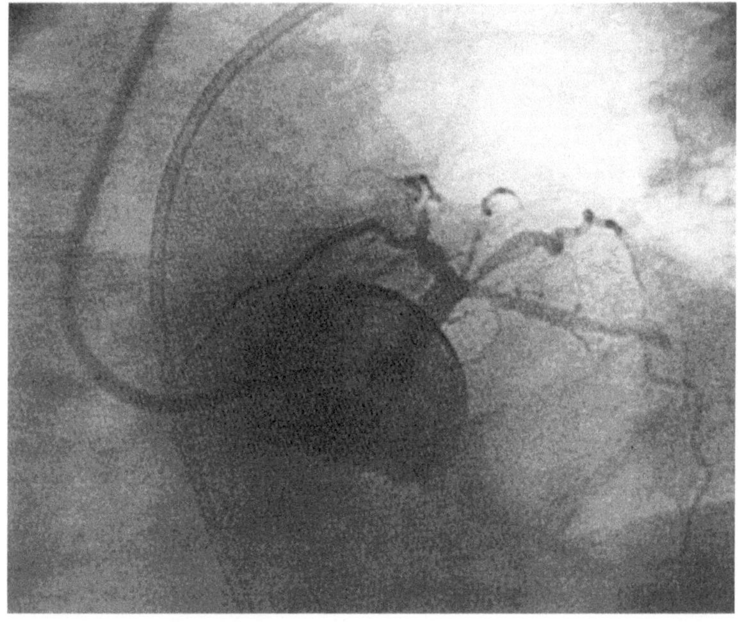

a

b

Fig. 1. Effects of "unsharp masking" on a digital angiogram of the left coronary artery with maximal KV-values. Recording angle: LAO 45°, Caudal 25°, a) unfiltered, b) filtered.

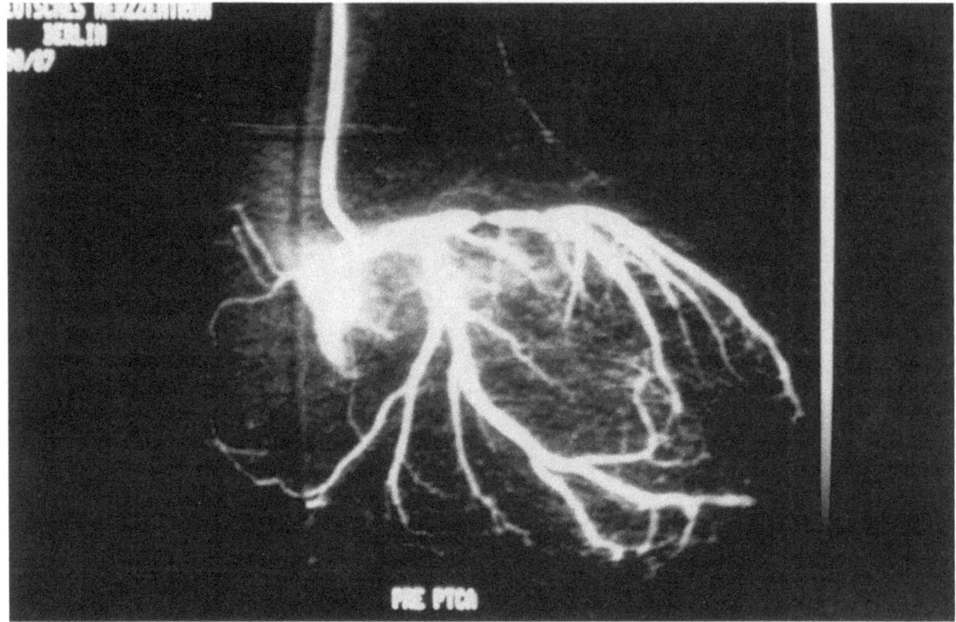

Fig. 2. Digital subtraction angiogram of a left coronary vessel. This quality of presentation even with ECG-triggering can hardly ever be reached.

Image quality

With real-time processing of images the recording image quality, as well as the fluoroscopic image quality, are essentially increased.

Availability of data

Immediately after acquisition the images are available for visual interpretation, as well as for computerized quantitative analysis.

Image acquisition and image quality

The digital acquisition runs simultaneously to normal cine acquisition modes and no additional handling is necessary. To receive optimal quality several image processing and enhancement techniques are involved, including contrast enhancement, contour enhancement, dynamic noise reduction, and gapfilling.

The latter has especially been shown to be useful, because the paradigma that lower image frequence acquisition is not possible in cardioangiography has changed. Even frequencies of 12.5 (15) frames per second produce excellent, flickerfree runs; therefore digital techniques use a lower effective total x-ray dose, since unchanged doses per frame are still required for adequate imaging.

18

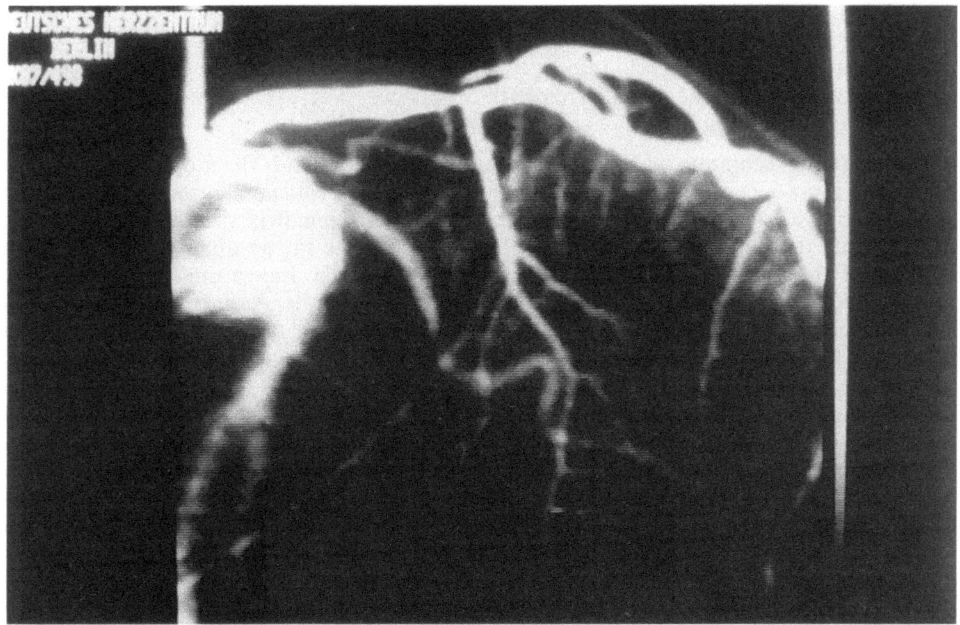

Fig. 3. Movement artefacts of the Ramus circumflexus and, at the same time, good presentation quality of the Ramus interventricularis anterior.

Availability of image data

One of the most important features that has strongly influenced the procedure in the cath-lab (in relation to performing an intervention during the same session in which the diagnostic catheter is performed) is the immediate availability of the images; the quality of these are comparable to cine. Every frame out of cine runs is excellent, with no blurring effects as are common in video still frames. The immediate redisplay of acquired images is not restricted to the last run. The storage capacity of adequate systems is within the range of a normal diagnostic investigation. The selection of the best roadmaps for various views of both planes is obvious.

In the predigital phase of coronary angiography the decision for an intervention was primarily based on visual inspection of the coronary anatomy. With the employment of digital systems these decisions can increasingly be based on objective quantitative values.

Digital fluoroscopy with high contrast gives dose-dependent access to picture quality which basically reaches angiography standards.

Digital angiography

Digital equipment uses all conventional components of the x-ray system [16]. The visible spectrum of light at the image intensifier exit comprises the basis for conventional film exposure as well as the on-line digitization of the video signal, which is enhanced with special filter techniques before being redisplayed. At the same time, digital images are available for quantitative analysis. The storage of the images on fast image discs provides the user with repeated display of image sequences or the selection of adequate still frames. In this context the following technical elements are of essential interest:

- x-ray technique (focus size, image intensifier, dose);
- image matrix size (spatial resolution);
- frame rate (temporal resolution);
- filter technique (image enhancement);
- storage technology.

In the analog technique, film quality, including development is the most critical issue in the image reproduction, whereas for digital imaging the problem can mostly be reduced to x-ray and video system parameters. The question of the matrix size (512^2 or 1024^2) is, disregarding the data processing effort, dependent on the image quality, which mainly consists of the modulation transfer function (MTF) of the image intensifier, the x-ray performance, the focus spot size, and the geometric conditions. An increase of resolution can only be reached in connection with an improvement of the MTF and not by just increasing the matrix size (which otherwise produces a subjectively better looking picture without increasing picture information content).

The image intensifier (with 9 resp. 6 inches) typically used in cardioangiography has a MTF that transfers frequences up to 4 lp/mm (the practical, usable frequency); however, it can cover 0 to 2 lp/mm, if the threshold is set at about 20% relative contrast [37]. A matrix with 512^2 image elements and a corresponding selection of the scanning window (overframing) reaches 2.2 lp/mm as border frequency. Extending to a larger matrix in connection with HDTV (high resolution video) will lead to a more homogeneous image impression.

For the subjective visual impression the filter technique is important. Unsharp masking leads to excellent image quality and is especially beneficial where vessels filled with contrast media can only be shown in a very diffuse manner, which occurs in extremly oblique projections that need high kV-value for imaging due to the large volume x-rayed (Fig. 1). The image enhancement techniques can also be used for fluoroscopy.

Digital subtraction angiography

Digital subtraction angiography (DSA) offers the basis to present anatomic relations and to quantify their functional effects [2, 22]. Since its introduction in clinical practice (1979/80) it has not gained importance for cardiac angiography. The reason for this is based on the complex motion of the heart, which makes adequate subtraction of congruent image pairs almost impossible. The few good examples that already exist are an exception (Fig. 2). In Fig. 3 movement artefacts can especially be recognized in the area of postero and lateral walls, even in correctly ECG-triggered projections (Fig. 3).

The DSA in the intra-arterial ECG-triggered form is best suited for diagnosis of large vessels like the aorta, extracranial vessels, etc. Common diagnostic questions like localization and geometry, as well as derived parameters concerning functional effects, e.g., vascularity of an organ or flow direction, can be adequately addressed and quantitatively evalutated [24] (Figs. 4 and 5). If the geometry within an image sequence has not changed, topography and function can be displayed in one frame. The information of a single pixel presents functional values, like starting time or maximum of contrast, which allows a rough estimation of flow [7, 8]. The use of DSA for diagnosis of congenital cardiac disorders, especially for the planning of surgical reconstruction, can be helpful if the structure's size and target exceed motion artefacts.

The main advantages arise for resolution- and function-dependent presentations. Even multiple runs, as, for example, are necessary to exactly locate a structure in its most appropriate projection, are possible since minimal amounts of contrast medium are needed. This can be of special interest in congenital cardiac disorders.

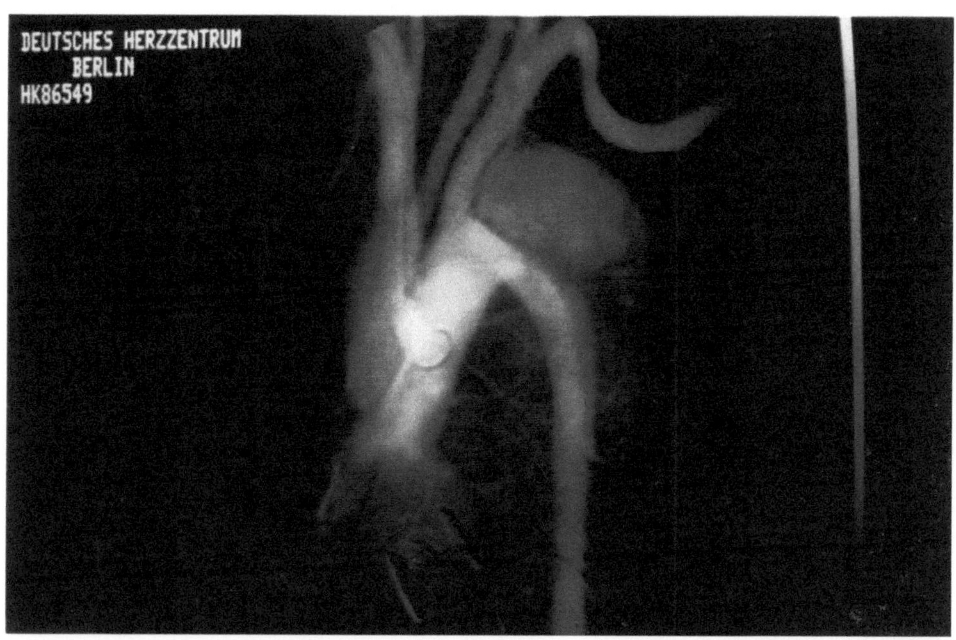

a

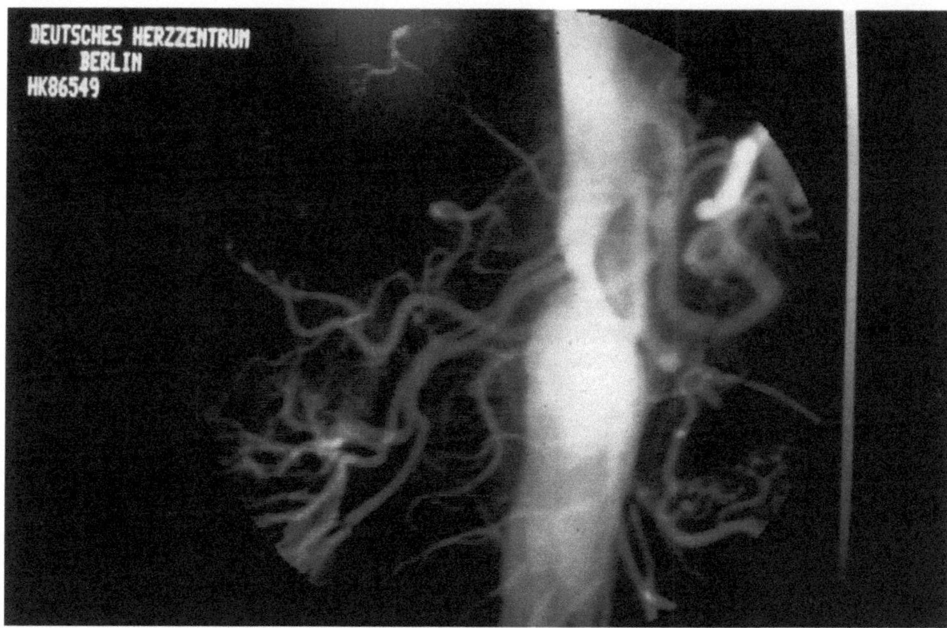

b

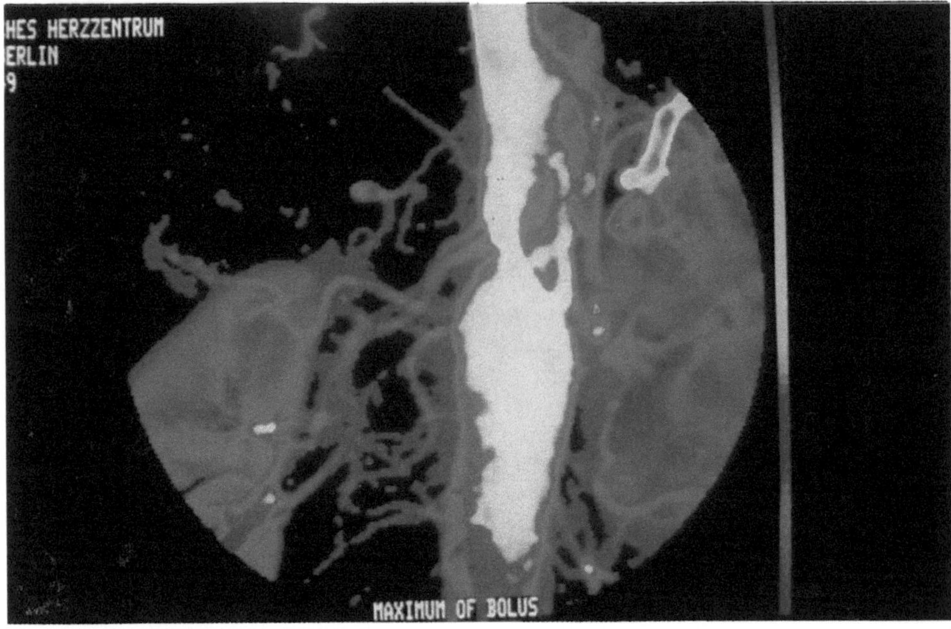

c

Fig. 4. Intra-arterial ECG-triggered DSA of an aortic aneurysm. The dissection starts in the aortic arch (4a) and ends on the same level of the renal arteria (4b). The question concerning the vascularity of the kidneys can be diagnosed with the help of a parameter image (4c), which represents the contrast media spreading in one image sequence.

Digital coronary angiography

In the last decade the importance of selective coronary angiography was heightened by the fact that not only changes of the coronary arteries are diagnosed [13], but also therapeutic interventions are supported [12]. The current numbers for this kind of therapy are presented in Fig. 6. These new treatment methods, however, have shown some essential drawbacks of the film-based conventional angiography. Especially the consequent application of coronary angioplasty immediately after a diagnostic catheterization requires a ready reproduction of image sequences without loss of quality. The common video technique does not deliver reasonable stillframes. The possibility to quantify distinct regions with objectivible methods during the examination is also not given, and the purely visual evaluation due to the high intra- and inter-observer variability is another well-known problem and, therefore, another error source in immediate decisions [21, 32, 38]. With the help of digital angiography solutions are available that include functional parameters like stenosis resistance, flow reserve or even flow distribution [1, 6].

Quantification

Information supplied by angiographic image sequences includes morphologic and functional components. The analysis – that is the method of information processing – can occur qualitatively or quantitatively. In conventional angiography the information supply is only evaluated qualitatively and mainly refers to the morphology. Functional parameters can also only be acquired qualitatively via mental integration of one or more image

22

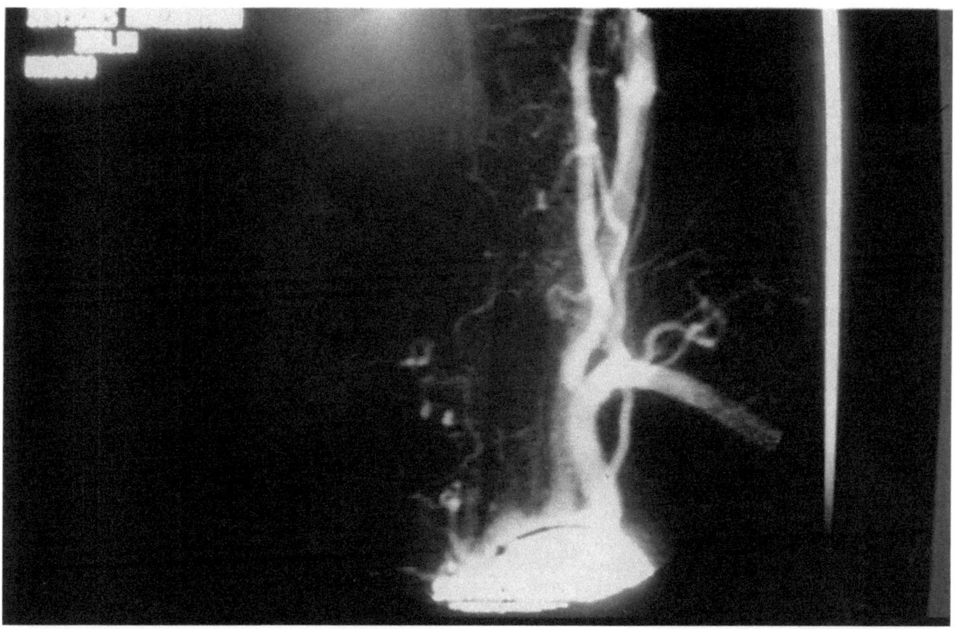

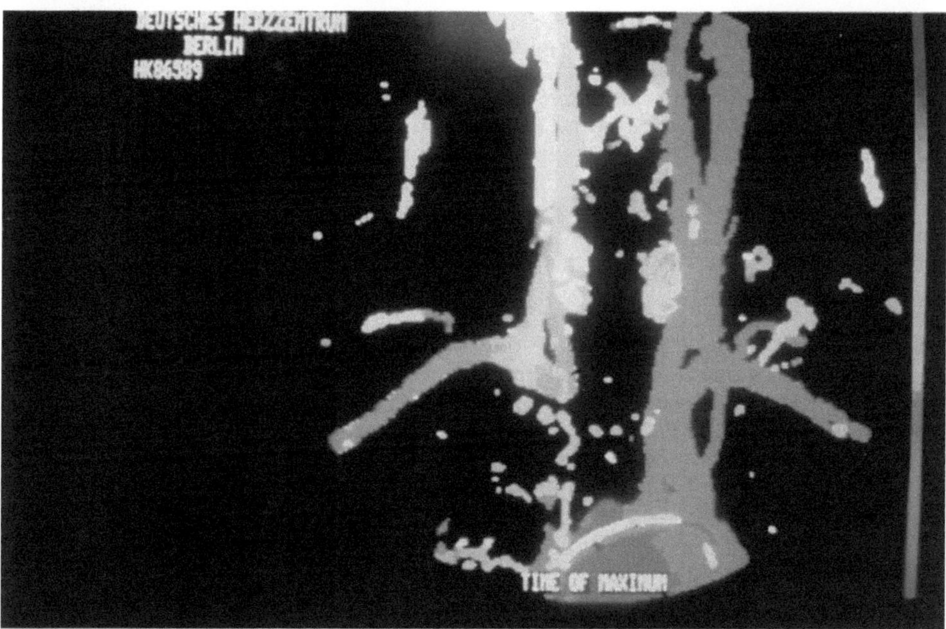

Fig. 5. Intra-arterial ECG-triggered DSA of a subclavian steal syndrome on the right side (5a). In the parameter image (5b) it can clearly be seen that blood resp. contrast medium flows to the head via the left Carotis interna and is supplied from the brain basis over the Carotis interna-right, the Arteria subclavia, and the Arteria vertebralis right (white). The arrival time is coded as color: blue = early, white = late.

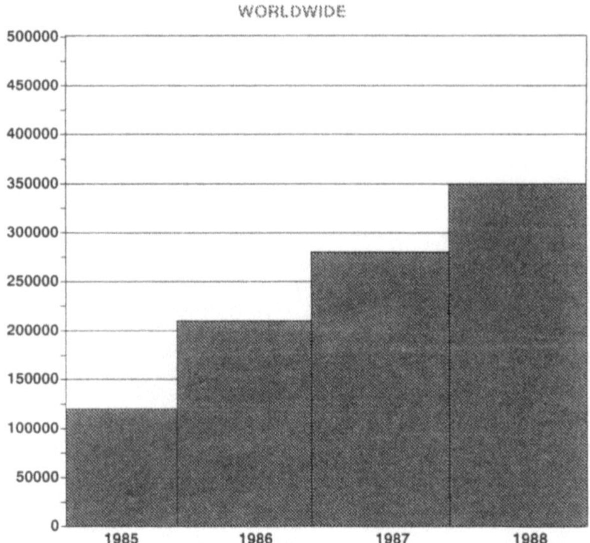

Fig. 6. Increasing numbers of PTCA worldwide/year.

sequences. Diagnostic decisions are based on a visual analysis of the distribution of the contrast medium. Alternatives to this situation, toward a more objective and thus reproducible evaluation are quantitative image analysis methods [27, 33, 35] using common models for volume, wall motion, and stenosis evaluation, and manually validated by well published studies. The methods applied are directly transferable into the complete analysis, which is based on digital images using internal reference points for adequate reliability (Fig. 7). The necessity to quantify coronary findings is not only due to the large variability of visual image interpretation, but especially to the functional aspects to the evaluation [9, 14, 15]. "Percent stenosis" by itself is not an exact description of the anticipated consequences of a narrowing. The functional relevance of the stenosis can be expressed by a complex parameter set that takes absolute diameter, form, and length of stenosis, as well as blood pressure and flow into consideration [20].

To meet these demands digital angiography not only requires excellent x-ray techniques, but also requires advanced techniques for image representation. The primary diagnosis algorithms, which extract a stenosed section of a vessel in a digital image, are based on edge-detection procedures and thus form the prerequisite for a detailed analysis [3, 18, 19, 28, 30]. Beginning with a starting point and an end point, the user indicates the section of vessel to be quantified, and an algorithm searches the median line. Orthogonally the density profile will be examined on both sides for possible vascular contour points. From phantom examinations it is known that the best contour point lies between the first and the second partial derivation of the density profile. These contour points are put together in a cost matrix to form a final contour line. Vessel ramifications can be recognized and, for subsequent treatment, can be recorded in a table [4]. Results of the automatic edge-detection are the contours of the selected coronary segments (Fig. 8); they form the basis for a detailed quantification, where obvious inaccuracies [29] can be corrected by interaction of the observer.

To improve the reliability of calculated geometric and hemodynamic parameters,

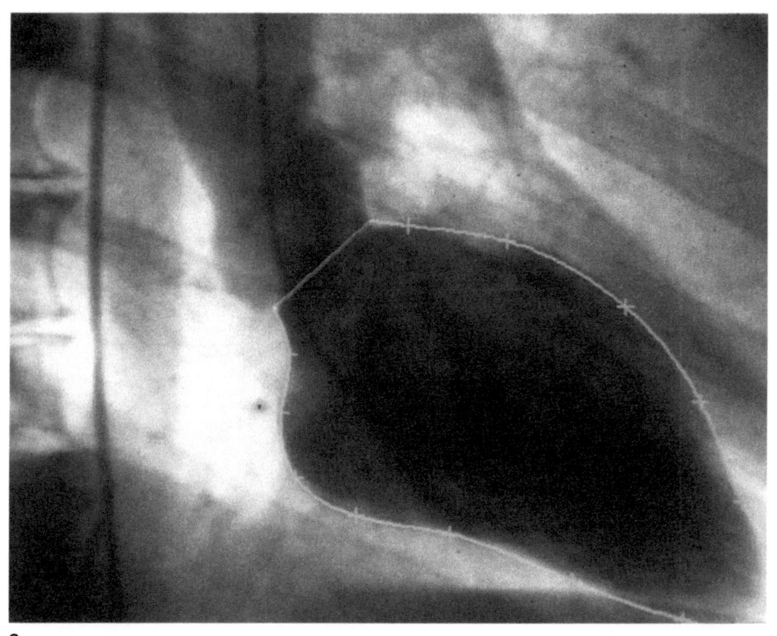

a

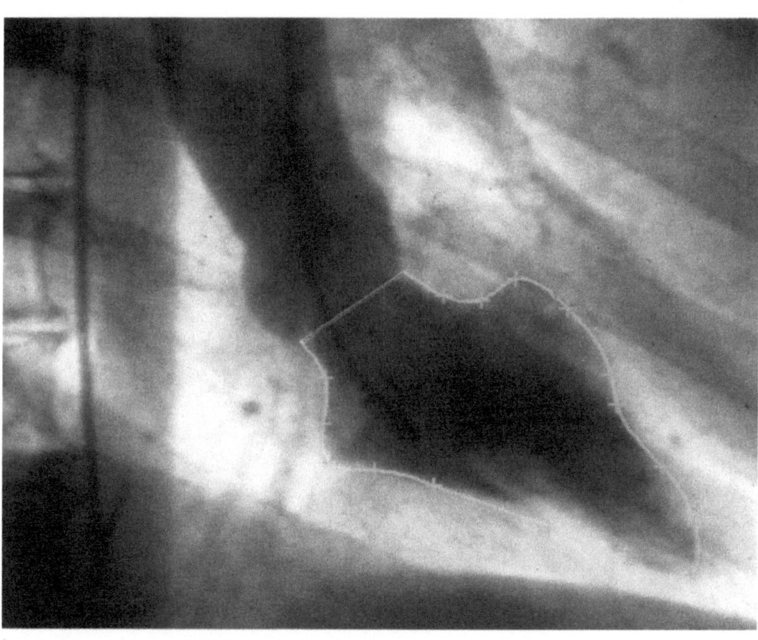

b

DIASTOLE
SYSTOLE
BIPLAN
RAO
LAO
EDV: SIMPSON   181.54   [ML]
ESV: SIMPSON   61.20   [ML]

c

REF   [CM]
PKT. 10   1.23
PKT. 20   0.73
PKT. 30   1.26
PKT. 40   1.06
PKT. 50   0.90
PKT. 60   0.52
PKT. 70   0.75
PKT. 80   0.92
PKT. 90   0.72
PKT. 100   -0.74
MOTIONS
AVERAGE   0.68

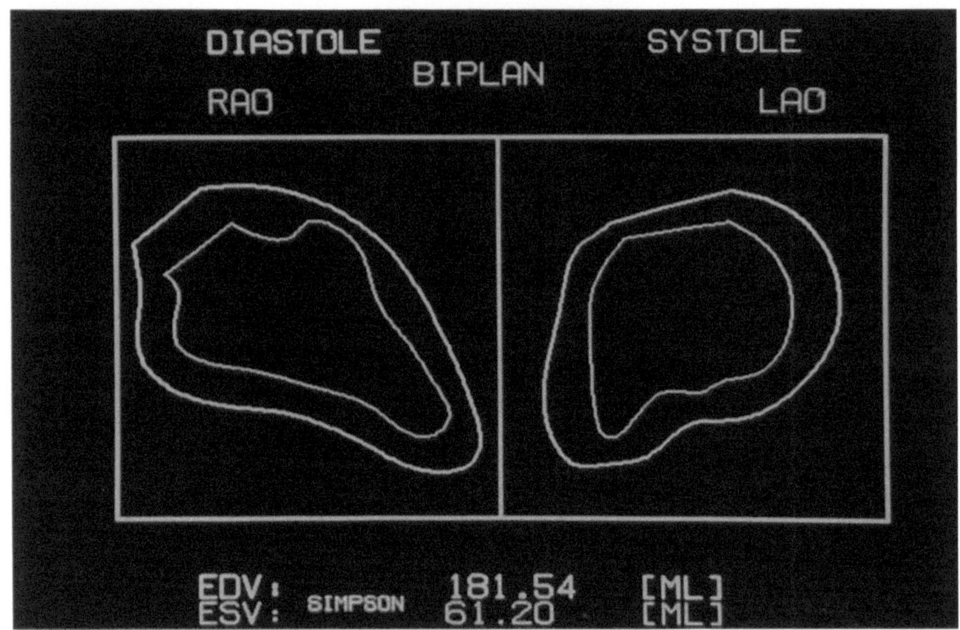

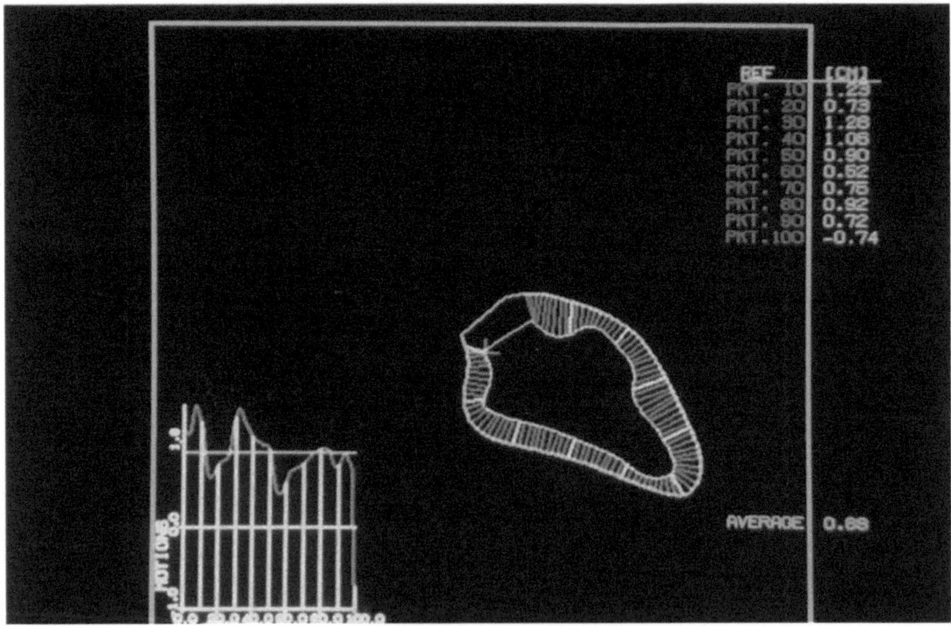

d

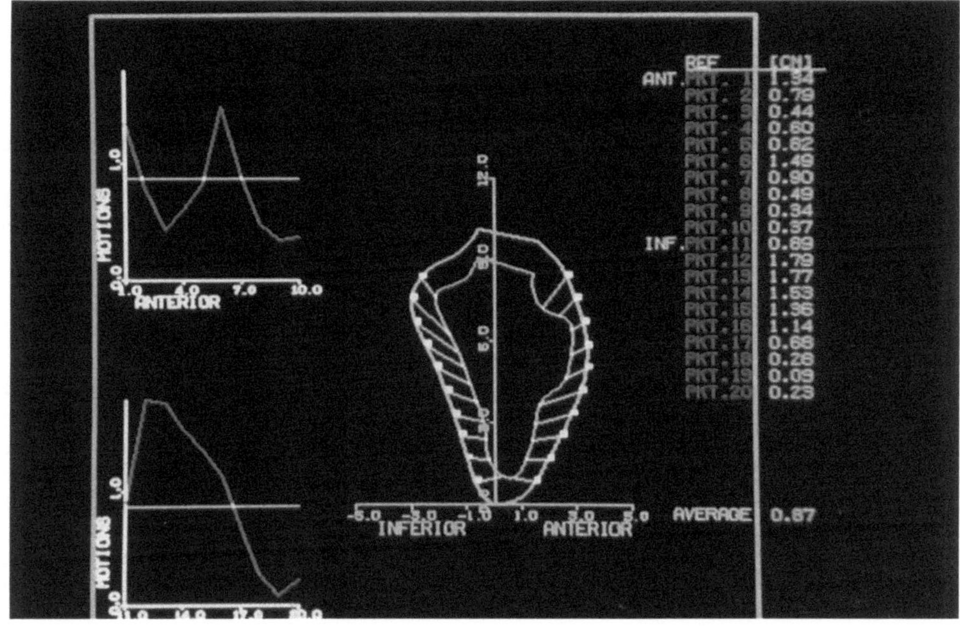

e

Fig. 7. Ventricle evaluation and wall-motion analysis. The input of a few points in diastole (7a) and systole (7b) is usually enough to receive exact contours by interpolation of cubic splines. Models of different complexity can be used for the calculation of the volume (7c). Adequate wall-motion models, e.g., according to models by Sheehan (7d) or Slager (7e) can be used. Image material: unfiltered original data recorded with 25 fr/s biplane on a Philips DCI.

different complex error calculations have to be included, such as corrections for pincushion distortion, magnification, and point spread function, by using deconvolution and densitometric functions.

Geometric correction

Pincushion distortion

The first step in geometric correction is the enhancement of the pincushion presentation error. The consequences of this error are rather small at the center of an image intensifier but increase toward the border. Digital systems display an additional distortion in a vertical direction that also has to be taken into account.

The systematic of the pincushion distortion does not correspond to a variable enlargement, which grows towards the edge [5, 17]. This radial distortion, which is described in the literature, is only one part of the pincushion distortion. Corresponding with models of the digital photogrammetry and remote sensing it is useful to use higher grade polynoms for rectification. In this way, a transformation T[f,g] is defined and the location coordinates of the original image O(x,y) are transformed into the location coordinates of the "enhanced" image B(x',y').

$$x' = f(x,y) = a_0 + a_1x + a_2y + a_3x^2 + a_4xy + a_5y^2 + \ldots$$

$$y' = g(x,y) = b_0 + b_1x + b_2y + b_3x^2 + b_4xy + b_5y^2 + \ldots$$

The recording of a regular raster with known grid size supplies the basis for a set of pass points to calculate such a polynom. The equation is solved by a best fit solution. For evaluation of the quality of the selected retification model the calculation of residuals is useful. The size and the direction of the deviation of the enhanced point to its ideal coordinates is measured and presentable (Fig. 8).

The application of the correction of the pincushion distortion either takes place for the whole image, which will be enhanced in a split second through the use of special image processors, or especially in quantitative analysis calculating only results, considering contour points of the coronary segment or of the ventricle with respect to their localization in the intensifier field.

Magnification

The goal of all quantifications in cardioangiography is the calculation of absolute parameter values like length, diameter or volume. To reach this, a relation between the real and the presented size must be found. For this, either sizes of known objects, like the catheter diameter [33], markers on the catheter or system parameters, like the distance between x-ray tube – patient – image intensifier are used. In monoplane systems this magnification factor is only valid in one layer, which is parallel to the image intensifier and where either the reference object or – when using system parameters – the virtual reference point is located. Upon the usage of biplane recordings and image plans that are orthogonal towards each other, the magnification factor for each point of the space, which is defined by the two images, is clearly calculable. The consequent use of biplane systems is a necessary precondition for maximum accuracy of the quantification. To establish the extent of orthogonality necessary model calculations and phantom measurements are currently conducted.

Point-spread function

The correlation of real-to-measured diameters of a phantom stenosis shows a non-linear relation: small diameters ($< 1.5\,$mm) are over-estimated and diameters smaller than $0.5\,$mm are presented at a constant value ($1.2\,$mm). This well-known phenomenon is due to the point-spread function of the x-ray imaging chain. For correction of this error an empirical correction function has proven useful especially for the quantitative evaluation of digitized film.

Adequate correction tables can also be prepared for digital on-line image sequences. The measured values are changed with the help of these correction regression, but the problem with diameters smaller than $0.5\,$mm remains unsolved. This can partly be overcome by incorporation of the densitometry [10, 11], which, however, cannot be put into action without supervision, but with its use error correction within these areas can be executed [25, 26].

Densitometric measurements are based on the fact that the brightness value resp. the gray level value within one pixel has a direct relation to the x-ray absorbed by the amount of dye [23, 31, 36]. The integral between the right and the left vessel contours of a gray value profile that is normally on the median line of the vessel is an index for the sectional area of the vessel at this location. The basic requirement for a quantitative measurement of these integrals is a quasi linearity of the system. For digitized films this assumption is not valid. On-line digital angiography systems, as they are presently available, provide stable conditions for densitometric evaluation.

Phantom measurements show that the densitometry, i.e., the gray value integrals over

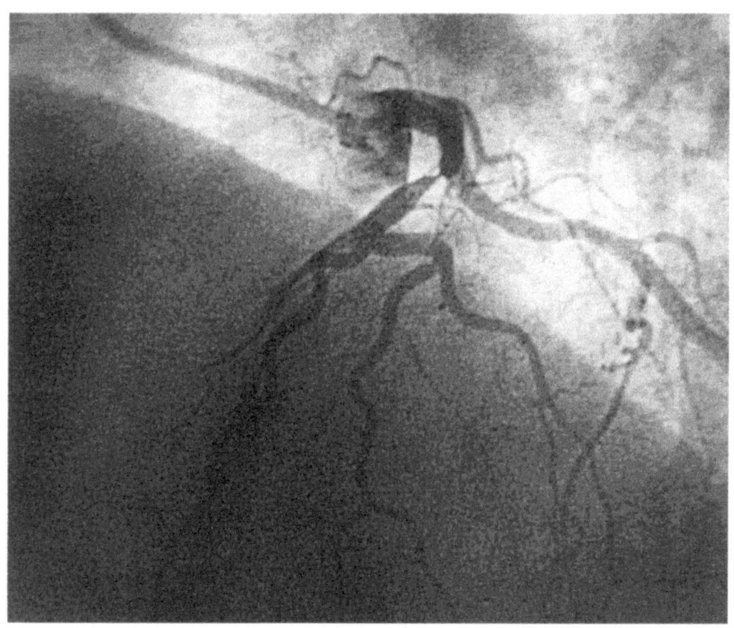

a

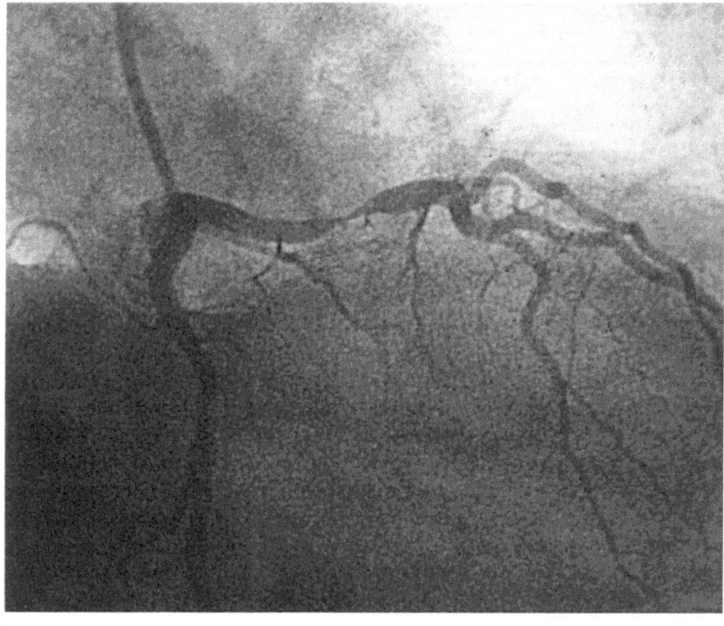

b

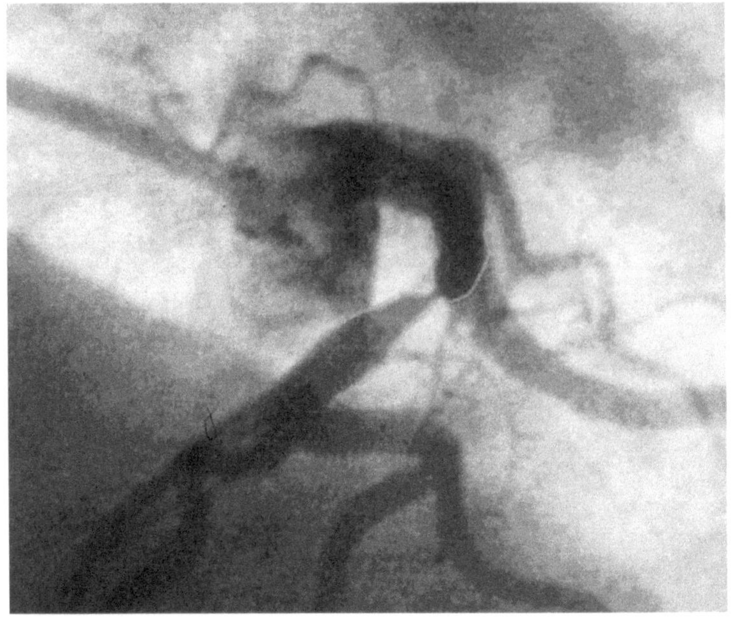

c

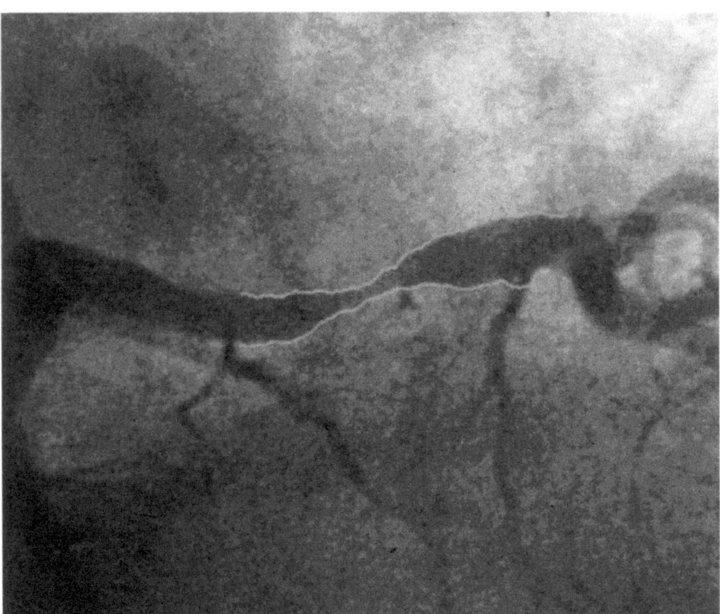

d

Fig. 8. Automatic contour recognition from digital biplane (orthogonal) coronary angiograms: 8a) LAO, 8b) RAO. 8c, 8d) zoomed images with contours.

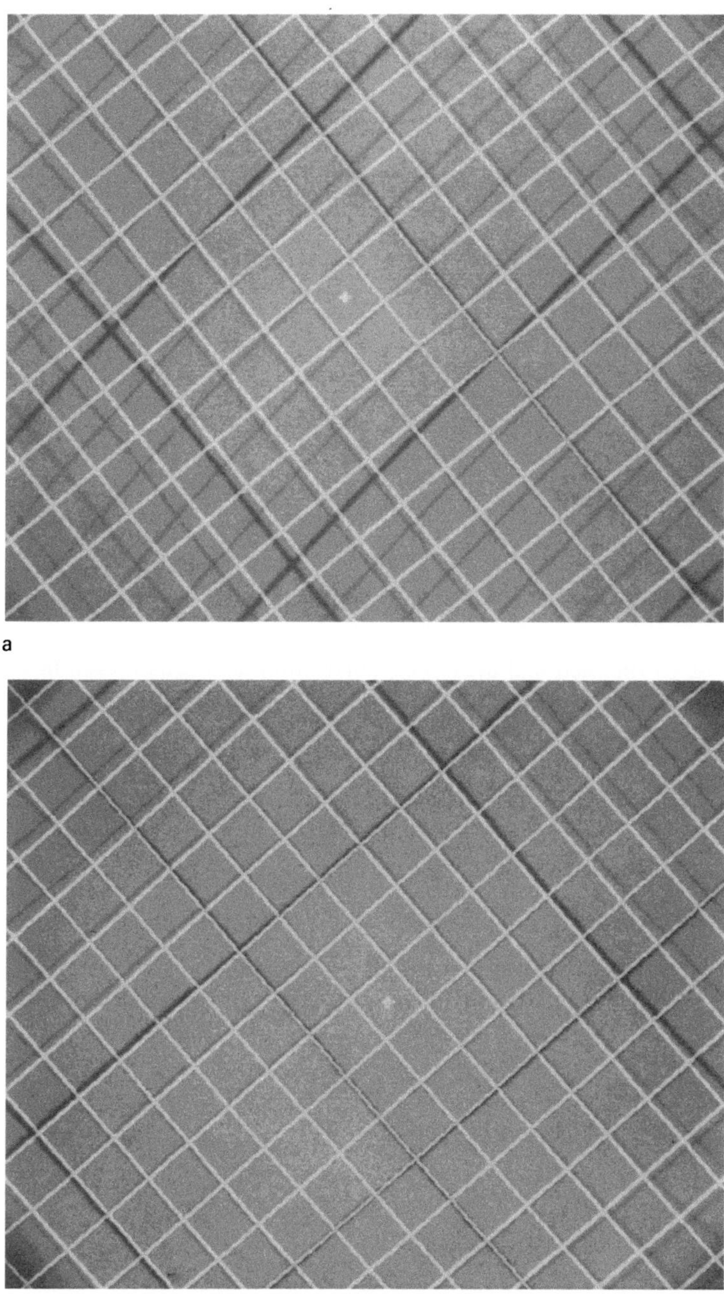

Fig. 9. Pincushion distortion: recording of a regular 1-cm raster with a DCI-System (Philips) overlapped with a synthetical raster (9a). Rectified image overlapped with a synthetic raster (9b).

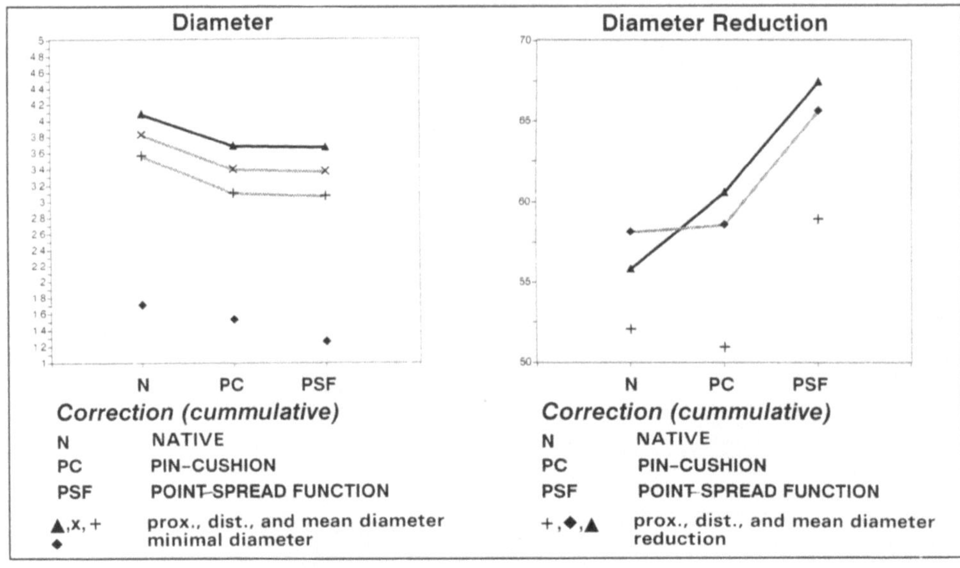

Fig. 10. Effects on diameter (9a) and diameter reduction (9b) cummulatively using correction procedures.

a profile, correlate close to the sectional area. This correlation is adequate even in the sub-millimeter range. Thus it is possile to execute an additional correction for the respective area of interest.

The relation between true (Dt) and measured (Dm) diameter and the corresponding density integrals D_1, D_2 is

$$\frac{D_1}{D_2} = \frac{c_1 * \left(\frac{Dt_1}{2}\right)^2 * \pi}{c_2 * \left(\frac{Dt_2}{2}\right)^2 * \pi}$$

For a limited area c_1 and c_2 are constant factors with $| c_1 - c_2 | < \varepsilon$.

With that the measurement accuracy for small diameters within the sub-millimeter area can be improved essential. The correction equation is

$$Dm_1 = \sqrt{\frac{D_1}{D_2}} * Dm_2,$$

where D_1 is the density integral of the small diameter, D_2 is that of a larger reference diameter Dm_2.

Measurement errors

Since the measurement error represents an inavoidable, but also calculable value, it can be integrated into the result [34] (Fig. 10). This is done with the help of error-spreading analyses that are carried out for all parameters, and which were derived from the measured values. Accuracy of measurements can thus be relativated and, for all parameters, expressed as a range of validity. The additional integration of clinical findings will further improve the usefulness of these corrected quantitative interventions.

32

References

1. Alderman EL, Berte LE, Harrison DC, Sanders W (1981) Quantitation of coronary artery dimensions using digital image processing. Proceedings of SPIE, Vol. 314, pp 273–278
2. Barrett W, Seibert T, Hines H (1984) Automated Detection of Coronary Arteries and Quantification of Percent Stenosis from DSA Images. Computers in Cardiology, pp 123–126
3. Beier J, Oswald H, Fleck E (1988) Erkennung und Quantifizierung von Koronarstenosen aus angiographischen Röntgenbildern. In H Bunke, O Kübler, P Stucki (Hrsg.): Mustererkennung 1988, 10. DAGM-Symposium, Zürich, Sept., Proceedings, Springer
4. Beier J, Oswald H, Fleck E (1988) Segmentierung von Gefäßverzweigungen aus angiographischen Röntgenbildern. In A Pinz (Hrsg): Wissensbasierte Mustererkennung, R Oldenburg Verlag Wien-München.
5. Brown BG, Bolson EL, Dogde HT (1986) Quantitative computer techniques for analyzing coronary arteriograms. In: Progress in Cardiovascular Diseases, Vol. 28, No. 6, pp 403–418
6. Brown BG, Bolson E, Frimer M (1977) Estimation of dimensions, hemodynamic resistance, and atheroma mass of coronary artery lesions using the arteriogram and digital computation. Circulation, Vol. 55, pp 329–337
7. Bürsch JH et al (1983) Myocardial perfusion studies by digital angiography computers in Cardiology. Long Beach, CA, IEEE Computer Society, 1983, pp 343–346
8. Bürsch JH et al (1983) Arterial blood flow analysis by digital angiography in Digital Imaging in Cardiovascular Radiology, PH Heintzen, R Brennecke (eds.) Stuttgart, Thieme, pp 115–123
9. Collins SM, Skorton DJ, Harrison DG, White CW (1982) Quantitative computerbased videodensitometry and the physiological significance of a coronary stenosis. Computers in Cardiolog, pp 229–222
10. Doriot PA, Pochon Y (1985) Densitometry of coronary arteries – an improved physical model. IEEE Computers in Cardiology, pp 91–94
11. Doriot PA, Honegger HP, Merier G (1981) Measurement of the Degree of coronary stenosis by digital Densitometry. Computers in Cardiology, p 329–332
12. Fleck E, Oswald H (1988) Digitales Röntgen in der Diagnostik und invasiven Therapie der koronaren Herzerkrankung, Röntgenstrahlen 59
13. Gensini GG (1975) Coronary arteriography. Futura Publishing Company
14. Gottwik MG, Siebes M, Kirkeiide RL (1984) Hämodynamik von Koronarstenosen. Zeitschrift für Kardiologie, Vol. 73, pp 47–54
15. Gould KL (1985) Quantification of coronary artery stenosis in vivo. Circulation Research, Vol. 57, pp 341–353
16. Grossmann, W (1986) Cardiac catheterization and angiography. Lea and Febinger, Philadelphia
17. Kirkeiide RL, Fung P, Smalling RW (1982) Automated evaluation of vessel diameter from arteriograms. Computers in Cardiology, pp 215–218
18. Kirkeiide RL, Wüsten B, Gottwick M (1981) Computer assisted evaluation of angio findings. In: Thrombose und Atherogenese, Pathophysiologie und Therapie der arteriellen Verschlußkrankheit, Verlag G. Witzstock, pp 414–417
19. LeFree MT, Simmon SB, Lewis RJ (1985) Digital Radiographic coronary Artery Quantification. Computers in Cardiology, pp 99–102
20. Logan SE (1975) On the fluid mechanics of human coronary artery stenosis. IEEE Transactions on biomedical engineering, pp 327–334
21. Meier B, Gruentzig AR, Pyle R (1983) Assessment of stenoses in coronary angioplasty, Inter- and intraobserver variability. International Journal of Cardiology, Vol. 3, pp 159–169
22. Moodie DS, Yiannikas J (1986) Digital Subtraction Angiography of the Heart and Lungs. Grune & Stratton, Inc.
23. Nichols AB, Christopher FO (1984) Quantification of relative coronary arterial stenosis by cinevideo densitometric analysis of coronary artiograms. Circulations, Vol. 69, pp 512–522
24. Obermöller U, Witte G, Höhne KH (1983) Parametrische Bilder aus intravenösen Angiogrammen des linken Herzventrikels. VDE-Fachberichte 35, Mustererkennung, VDE-Verlag GmbH, pp 47–53
25. Oswald H, Fleck E, Beier J (1987) Densitometric correction of vessel diameter from digital arteriograms. In GH Schneider, E Vogler (Hrsg.): Digitale bildgebende Verfahren – Interventionelle Verfahren – Integrierte digitale Radiologie, Springer Verlag, Berlin/New York
26. Oswald H, Beier J, Fleck E (1988) Densitometrisch korrigierte Gefäßdurchmesser in der digitalen Koronarangiographie. In E Fleck (Hrsg.): Koronare Herzerkrankung und dilatative Kardiomyopathie: Diagnostik und Therapie, MMW

27. Reiber JHC, Serruys PW, Slager CJ (1986) Quantitative Coronary and left Ventricular Cineangio-
    graphie. Martinus Nijhoff Publisher, Boston/Dordrecht/Lancaster
28. Reiber JHC, Kooijman CJ, Slager CJ (1985) A novel approach to the accurate assessment of coronary
    arterial dimensions from cineangiograms. Diagnostic Imaging, pp 87–89
29. Reiber JHV, Serruys PW, Kooijmann CJ (1985) Assessment of short- medium-, and long-term
    variations in arterial dimensions. Circulations, Vol. 71, pp 280–288
30. Reiber JHC, Kooijmann CJ, Slager CJ (1984) Coronary artery dimensions from cineangiograms –
    methodology and validation of a computer-assisted procedure. IEEE Transactions on medical
    imaging, pp 131–141
31. Reiber JHC, Troost GJ, Gerbrands JJ (1981) Densitometric Assessment Severity of coronary Obstruc-
    tion from monoplane views. Computers in Cardiology, pp 333–336
32. SanMarco M, Brooks S, Blankenhorn D (1978) Reproducibility of a consensus panel in the interpreta-
    tion of coronary angiograms. American Heart Journal, Vol. 96, pp 430–437
33. Siebes M, Selzer RH (1985) How accurate is the catheter as a reference for arterial dimensions in
    quantitative coronary angiography? IEEE Computers in Cardiology, pp 9–14
34. Siebes M, Lenzen H, Gottwik (1983) Influence of geometric Errors in quantitative Angiography on the
    Evaluation of stenotic Hermodynamics. Computers in Cariology, pp 385–388
35. Spears JR, Sandor T, Als AV (1983) Computerized image analysis for quantitative measurement of
    vessel diameter from cineangiograms. Circulations, Vol. 68, pp 453–461
36. Tobis J et al (1987) Videodensitometric Determination of Minimum Coronary Artery luminal
    Diameter before and after Angioplasty. America Journal of Cardiology, Vol. 59, pp 38–44
37. Verhoeven LAJ (1985) Digital Subtraction Angiography (DSA) – the technique and an analysis of the
    physical factors influencing the image quality. Dissertationsschrift der Technischen Hochschule Delft
38. Zir LM et L (1976) Interobserver Variability in Coronary Angiography. Circulations, Vol. 53, pp 627–
    632

Author's address:
Prof. Dr. E. Fleck
Klinik für Innere Medizin – Kardiologie
Deutsches Herzzentrum Berlin
Augustenburger Platz 1
1000 Berlin 65, FRG

Do Long-term Inflations Reduce the Occurrence of Acute Complications after Coronary Balloon Angioplasty?

W. Rutsch and H. Schmutzler

Abteilung für Innere Medizin mit Schwerpunkt Kardiologie und Pneumologie (Leiter: Prof. Dr. H. Schmutzler) Universitätsklinikum Rudolf-Virchow, Berlin, FRG

Introduction

Balloon angioplasty has become a very successful technique for treatment of coronary artery disease, providing high angiographic and clinical success rates. Limitations of procedures include inadequate dilatation, acute complications such as abrupt closure, acute myocardial infarction, emergency bypass surgery, and death, as well as chronic restenosis. From the procedural standpoint rapid development of chest pain limits balloon angioplasty of proximal stenoses with large regions of myocardium at risk. In most clinical institutions, balloon angioplasty procedures must be kept under 60 s in duration to avoid significant transmural myocardial ischemia, severe angina pectoris, arrhythmias, or a drop in aortic pressure. However, there is suggestive evidence that prolonged inflations of narrowed vascular segments may improve the rate of acute angiographic complications like dissections and abrupt closure, and reduce the chronic restenosis rate as well. An autoperfusion catheter system that allows myocardial perfusion during balloon inflation provides a number of significant advantages, including practically unlimited duration of inflations without angina, improved angiographic and clinical primary success rates, and a wide margin of safety in cases of acute occlusion requiring emergency bypass surgery. The autoperfusion catheter allows clinically significant ongoing blood flow during balloon inflation in both animal and preliminary studies in humans [1]. Inflation with the STACK autoperfusion catheter was maintained for at least 30 min in animal experiments. The resulting prolonged vessel wall ischemia and subsequent damage could potentially create a scarred segment of coronary vessel, which might participate less in the complex proliferative processes that lead to restenosis [1].

Patients and methods

The STACK autoperfusion catheter (Advanced Cardiovascular Systems, Inc., Santa Clara, California, USA) allows blood to enter through proximal side holes, pass through a central lumen in the balloon, and exit through distal side holes so as to provide continuous distal coronary perfusion during PTCA. The catheter is a 3.7 F catheter with 14 side holes arranged in a linear pattern over the distal 10 cm of the catheter. Four of these side holes are located distal to the 2-cm long angioplasty balloon segment. The large internal diameter permits use of a 0.018-inch guidewire. After the balloon has crossed the site of the obstruction, the wire is then withdrawn so that it lies proximal to the side holes in order to allow continuous perfusion during balloon inflation. In vitro flow-rate specification provided by the manufacturer demonstrates sufficient flow at different pressure levels with different catheter sizes. Depending on the balloon size, an inflation pressure of 80 mm HG allows a blood flow of 70.4 ml/min (2.5 mm) and 63.9 ml/min (3.5 mm), respectively. The catheter material PE 600, a tapered shaft, and microglide surface coating give the catheter sufficient characteristics for use even in complicated coronary anatomy.

Table 1. Patients, Baseline characteristics (n = 63).

Mean age (years)	57.3 ± 9.4
Women	24%
Stable angina pectoris	81%
Unstable angina pectoris	17%
Acute myocardial infarction	2%
Vessel disease	
single	51%
double	32%
triple	17%
Previous myocardial infarction	50%

Single dilatations lasting more than 30 min were attempted. Angioplasty was considered angiographically successful when residual stenosis was less than 50%, and a clinical success was defined as residual stenosis of less than 50% without myocardial infarction, emergency bypass surgery or death. Although we initially limited use of the system to treatment of proximal lesions, primarily of the LAD and RCA and high-risk cases, increased experience led us to use this equipment as our first choice in the treatment of most atherosclerotic lesions, except with a vessel diameter of less than 2.5 mm. Inflation pressure of 7 atmospheres was standard, although the balloons can be inflated to 10 atmospheres without loss of autoperfusion characteristics.

Results

Since July 1989 we have employed the STACK autoperfusion catheter in 63 cases. The baseline characteristics of the study group is shown in Table 1. 8% of patients underwent angioplasty for treatment of restenosis after previous PTCA. 46% of patients had normal ECG findings, 20% had signs of anterior infarction, 30% inferior infarction, and 12% non-diagnostic ST-T changes associated with bundle-branch block that did not permit a diagnosis of transmural infarction. The distribution of lesions attempted was: segment 1, 3%; segment 2, 13%; segment 3, 11%; segment 4, 1%, segment 6, 32%; segment 7, 21%; segment 9, 2%; segment 11, 5%; segment 13, 8%; segment 14, 4%. A total of 76 lesions in 70 vessels were treated in 63 patients, with an average of 1.2 dilatations per patient. The stenoses were described as single discrete in 43% of patients, as tubular in 35%, and as stenoses with diffuse irregularities in 19% of patients. Complete coronary occlusion was present in three cases. 35% of patients had eccentric lesions with wide or narrowed bases. Side branches were present within the stenosis or the area of balloon in all but 23% of patients, and side branches were directly involved in the lesions in 35% of cases. 20% of stenoses were located in curves greater than 45° (Table 2). Procedural details by lesions are listed in Table 3.

Table 2. Characteristics of the lesions (n = 75).

Single discrete	43%
Multiple discrete	7%
Tubular	35%
Diffuse	19%
Total occlusion	3%
Eccentric geometry	35%
Branch point	77%
Bendpoint > 45°	20%

Table 3. Procedural details by lesion.

Balloon catheter diameter (mm)	2.5	45 (60%)
	3.0	23 (31%)
	3.5	7 (9%)
Number of inflations	mean	2.4 ± 1.7
	range	1–11
Total inflation time (s)	mean	1090 ± 800
	range	600–3600
Maximum inflation pressure (atm)	man	7.5 ± 2.0
	range	6–10

Total duration of inflation was 10 min in 7% of cases, 20 min in 41% of patients, and more than 30 min in the remaining 33% of cases. Satisfactory angiographic results were achieved with a single dilatation in 32%, with two inflations in 33%, and with three or more dilatations in 32%. Balloon angioplasty was terminated when severe chest pain developed. This was accompanied by significant ST-segment depression in the majority of patients. A significant fall in aortic pressure or severe arrhythmia did not require termination of angioplasty in any case. Angina developed rapidly in patients with large side branches located within the area occluded by the balloon catheter. In a few cases myocardial ischemia was related to narrow diameter of the coronary artery. Before angioplasty the mean degree of stenosis was 84 ± 9%, as compared to 30 ± 19% after treatment.

The primary angiographic success rate per patient with a residual stenosis of less then 50% in all segments attempted was 96%, and the clinical success rate was 95% (Table 4). Angiographic evaluation demonstrated no pathological findings in the dilated segments in 91% of patients, while intraintimal filling defects parallel to the lumen were visible during contrast administration in 5%. Dissection of the vessel wall with persistent contrast depots was found in 3.2% of patients. Coronary perfusion was not affected. Two patients with dilations lasting more than 30 min experienced dissection causing occlusion requiring emergency bypass grafting. One patient died of sepsis 10 days after surgery. In one patient attempted PTCA of the LAD resulted in occlusion of the circumflex artery. It was not possible to reestablish satisfactory perfusion, and the patient suffered an inferior infarction despite the use of the STACK autoperfusion catheter. The apparent cause was occlusive dissection, and we did not consider this a complication of dilatation with this device. We observed a total of two dissections with subsequent occlusion in 74 dilated segments. In both cases prolonged angioplasty did not produce a satisfactory result, and surgical revascularization was necessary.

Discussion

Standard balloon coronary angioplasty is limited by an abrupt closure rate of approximately 5% and a restenosis rate of approximately 30%. The STACK autoperfusion balloon

Table 4. Acute complications and success rates.

	in Pts.	(= %)
Abrupt closure	2	3.2
Myocardial infrction	1	1.6
Emergency CABG	2	3.2
Death	1	1.6
Angiographic success	72/75	96
Clinical success	60/63	95

catheter represents a significant advance in conventional balloon angioplasty. It allows clinically significant ongoing blood flow during balloon inflation. Erbel et al. [2] first reported the use of a coronary angioplasty catheter capable of passive perfusion of blood during balloon inflation. Turi et al [3] recently reported on experimental results of a different passive perfusion balloon catheter. In this study, radioactive microspheres were used to measure myocardial blood flow during angioplasty. These data showed significant improvement of flow compared with standard angioplasty. Longer duration of inflation probably contributes to improved angiographic and clinical success rates and may influence the rate of chronic restenosis. The major advantages of the autoperfusion catheter demonstrated in this pilot study were freedom from chest pain during inflation, a low rate of acute complications, and a wide margin of safety due to maintenance of myocardial perfusion in cases of occlusion requiring emergency bypass surgery. The new catheter material PE 600, the microglide coating, and the tapered shaft have broadened the catalogue of indications for angioplasty. Practically all relevant segments of the coronary vasculature can be reached with this catheter system. The STACK autoperfusion catheter is limited by its larger deflated profile and does not prevent significant ischemia if the dilated lesion is located near a major side branch that is occluded by the balloon during inflation.

References

1. Stack RS, Quigley PJ, Collins G, Phillips III HR (1988) Perfusion balloon catheter. Am J Cardiol 61: 776–80G.
2. Erbel R, Clas W, Busch U, von Seelen W, Brennecke R, Blömer H, Meyer J. New balloon catheters for prolonged percutaneous transluminal coronary angioplasty and bypass flow in occluded vessels. Cathet Cardiovasc Diagn 1986; 12: 116–123.
3. Turi ZG, Campbell CA, Gottimukkala MV, Kloner RA. Preservation of distal coronary perfusion during prolonged balloon inflation with an autoperfusion angioplasty catheter. Circulation 1987; 6: 1273–1280.

Authors' address:
PD Dr. W. Rutsch
Universitätsklinikum Rudolf-Virchow
Freie Universität Berlin
Spandauer Damm 130
1000 Berlin 19, FRG

"High-risk" PTCA. Definition, Results, and Recommendations

G. O. Hartzler

Kansas City, Missouri, USA

Introduction

Since experience with different forms of invasive cardiologic treatment is increasing, it is necessary to optimize the indications for each technique. PTCA is the most widely used technique for reducing coronary artery stenoses; experience with the procedure has been garnered since the late 1970s.

There are risks with coronary angioplasty in several instances: first, immediate procedural risks consisting of morbitity and mortality from the invasive treatment itself. These risks are highly dependent on the patient, his medical precondition, and especially, the extent of impaired cardiac function. Secondly, there is the risk of the procedure to be unsuccessful, thus not leading to the desired therapeutic aim. Finally, the risk of unfavorable late outcome despite successful PTCA must be considered.

The task of this paper is to define criteria under which PTCA could be attempted despite increased risks. Criteria depend on the patient, the angioplaster, and the pecularities of the procedure. This paper deals with patient-dependent and procedural risks of coronary angioplasty.

Patient-dependent risk factors include:
- advanced age;
- poor LV function;
- prior bypass-surgery.

Procedural risk factors include:
- PTCA of left main coronary artery;
- PTCA in acute myocardial infarction;
- multilesion PTCA.

For this paper, 8000 PTCA procedures were evaluated. All risk factors mentioned above were found in a considerable number of cases. The exact figures are shown in Table 1.

PTCA of left main coronary artery

In 7000 procedures from May 1981 to December 1987, 100 patients (pts.) (= 1.4%; gender: 83/17 male/female; age: *m* 63 years, range 36–87 years) were treated with angioplasty of LMCA. Of them, 71 had "protected" angioplasty in LMCA, 29 were "unprotected". In this sample (number of procedures: 117), incidences of the other risk factors mentioned above were

age > 70 years	20%;
LV-EF < 40%	21%;
prior CABG	79%;
multilesion PTCA	78%.

Of the LMCAs, 110 (= 94%) could be dilated; 216/233 of the vessels in multilesion-cases (= 93%) could be successfully treated. Urgent CABG-surgery was necessary in two cases (= 1.7%); five patients died (= 4.3%).

Table 1. Factors for increased PTCA risks.

Risk factors	n	= %
Age > 70 years	1479	18
Poor LV function	1104	14
Prior bypass surgery	1561	19
Left main PTCA	138	1.7
PTCA in acute infarction	815	10
Multilesion PTCA	4601	58

Late results and follow-up data (with comparison of survival in "protected" and "unprotected" LMCA-cases) are given in Tables 2–3, and in Fig. 1.

These data can be compared with data of the CASS-study, concerning the outcome after different forms of treatment (1, 7).

The patients with Left-Main-Equivalent involvement in coronary artery disease in this study have been evaluated, data again were compared with those of the CASS-study, respectively (Table 4).

Based on the experience from these samples, the following recommendations concerning PTCA of LMCA should be observed (5, 11):
– if bypass surgery is possible, avoid PTCA;
– if the left main coronary artery is unprotected, which means inadequate blood supply by collaterals and/or patent bypass grafts, intraaortic balloon-pulsation or perfusion-systems should be used;
– dilate RCA stenoses first;
– dilate left graft stenoses first;
– observe systemic pressure and heart rate;
– shorter balloon inflation-times should be used, as dictated by hemodynamic response*;
– incremented balloon pressures and sizes should be used, avoiding over-expansion*.
*The two latter might be changed by using perfusion-balloons.

PTCA in patients with poor left-ventricular function

Our follow-up data (mean period 31 months) show survival-rates of the first, second, and third postoperative years of 74%, 72%, and 70% of patients, respectively indicating that the most dangerous phase is the immediate post-procedural period. Separating patients by more and less than 30% LV-ejection fraction, overall survival in the first group is 78%, in the latter, 37%.

The following recommendations should be observed:
– LV-function should be optimized before PTCA;

Table 2. LMCA-PTCA: Adverse procedural outcome; influence of "Protection".

Cardiac events	Total		"Protected"	"Unprotected"	Sign
	n	%	n	n	p <
Infarction	6	7	4	2	ns
Bypass surgery	13	14	7	6	0.01
Repeat PTCA	26	29	20	6	ns
Repeat LM-PTCA	4	15	10	4	ns
Total deaths	24	24	7	17	0.0005

Table 3. LMCA-PTCA: Follow-up data.

Outcome	CASS surgical	Study "protected"	Study "unprotected"
Procedural mortality	2.8–9.6%	2.4%	9%
Late survival (2 years)	88–93%	91%	45%

- β-blockers should be discontinued, dextran should be avoided;
- intra-aortic balloon pump should be prepared, resp., installed;
- low-osmolality contrast agent should be used; (non-ionics?);
- PTCA should be limited to critical stenoses in major vessels, if the patient is hemodynamically unstable;
- chronic total occlusions should be ignored, given sufficient time; contrast-medium load and patient tolerance are questionable.

PTCA in multiple-vessel disease

We have evaluated 6500 procedures of PTCA with the other high-risk subsets excluded. Excluded were patients over 70 years of age, with poor left-ventricular function, acute myocardial infarction, and LMCA-stenoses (procedures). The procedural outcome is shown in Table 5.

Since the results shown in Table 5 do not indicate that there is an increased risk of the procedure when dilating more than one lesion or more than one vessel. The following recommendation should be observed for cases with multilesion-PTCA [2, 3, 5, 6]:
- most significant stenoses should be dilated first; criteria of significance are the amount of myocardium at risk and the technical difficulties of the dilation;
- reasons for the preferential treatment of total occlusions and lesser significant stenoses are a low risk and a potential to provide collaterals, and a potential to increase stability in presence of complication with another artery at higher risk;
- proximal stenoses should be dilated before distal stenoses;
- Procedure should be stopped and staging should be performed if there is an unsatisfactory result with the initial stenoses.

PTCA in patients with advanced age

In our series there were 86 procedures undertaken in 75 patients aged 80–92 years. Many of them had several other risk factors for PTCA; including: unstable angina 57%; acute

Table 4. LMCA-PTCA.

Outcome	CASS surgical	CASS medical	This study (PTCA)
Procedural infarction	4.1%		1.3%
Procedural death	3.1%		2.5%
Survival: 1 year	95%	84%	90%
2 years	93%	73%	88%
3 years	91%	67%	88%

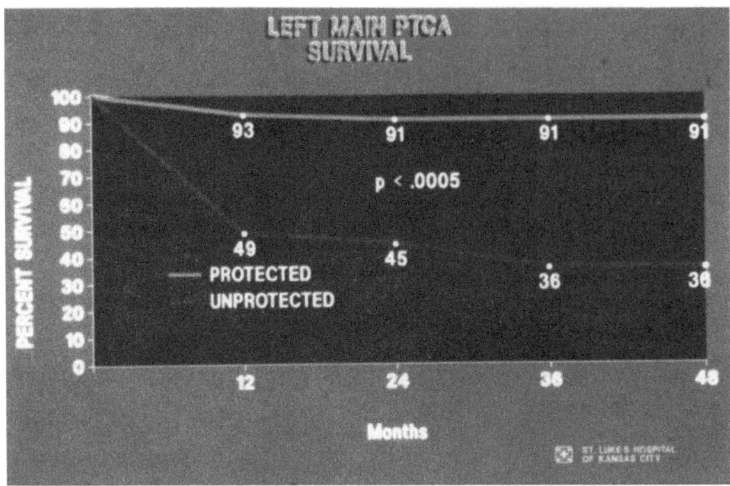

Fig. 1. Follow-up survival rates of PTCA of left main coronary artery (n = 117), distinguished between "protected" and "unprotected" LMCA-cases.

infarction 16%; prior bypass surgery 4%; poor LV function 15%; multivessel CAD 70%; multivessel PTCA 59%.

Primary success was achieved in 89%, one patient suffered acute myocardial infarction, and three patients died. In none was CABG surgery necessary.

In comparison, mortality-numbers in several publications (from 1973 to 1984) concerning death after bypass surgery in patients over the age of 70, range from 0% (in 25 pts.) to 22% (in 95 pts.) [10].

Late result data in those very elderly patients show an actuarial survival ratio of 77% after 1 year and 75% after 2 years (data of 70 patients).

Indications for intra-aortic balloon-pump

Prophylactic IABP should be installed under the following conditions:
– poor LV function (< 20–30%);
– in PTCA of "unprotected" LMCA;
– in PTCA of the single remaining artery or graft;
– in persisting arterial hypotension;
– in cases of acute infarct interventions, particularly in anterior MI with high LV-EDP and ejection fraction < 30%.

In summary, the following "Axioms" must be observed in case of "high-risk"-PTCA [5]:

Table 5. PTCA in multiple-vessel disease.

Outcome	Single-vessel-PTCA n = 1831	Multiple-vessel-PTCA n = 2385
Success	88%	96%
Death	5, = 0.3%	5, = 0.2%

Table 6. Risk ratio of PTCA according to subgroups.

Risk factor	No. n	Success %	Death %	Risk ratio*
LMCA-procedure	103	92	3.9	5.9
LMCA-equivalent-proced.	77	95	2.6	3.8
LV-EF < 40%	664	93	2.7	5.9
Age > 70 years	1038	94	1.4	2.6
All 3 vesels	305	97	1.3	1.9
Unstable angina	193	96	1.5	2.2

*determined by logistic regression analysis, holding all other factors constant.

- the management strategy must be individualized for each patient;
- the procedural goal (complete revascularization or palliation) should be determined in advance;
- full discussion with patient and family should be achieved in cases of elective procedure;
- surgical opinion should be considered;
- increased surgical preparedness should be achieved;
- technically complex PTCA is not equivalent to "high-risk" PTCA;
- multiple-vessel PTCA is not equivalent to "high-risk" PTCA;
- "high-risk" PTCA must be limited to advanced angioplasters only.

Assuming an experienced and competent angioplaster, the "risk" of PTCA is largely determined by associated factors of poor LV function, age, acute myocardial infarction, and intended left main coronary artery or equivalent dilatation.

References

1. Chaitman BR, Davis KB, Kaiser GL, Mudd G, Wiens RD, Ng CS, Passamani ER, Killip T (1986) The Role of Coronary Bypass Surgery for "Left Main Equivalent" Coronary Disease: the Coronary Artery Surgery Study Registry. Circulation 74 Suppl. III:17–25.
2. Dorros G, Lewin RF, Janke L (1987) Multiple Lesion Transluminal Coronary Angioplasty in Single and Multivessel Coronary Artery Disease: Acute Outcome and Long-Term Effect. J. Am Coll Cardiol 10:1007–13.
3. Dorros G, Stertzer SH, Cowley MJ, Myler RK (1984) Complex Coronary Angioplasty: Multiple Coronary Dilatations, AM J Cardiol 53 Suppl. C: 126C–130C.
4. Hartzler GO, Rutherford BD, McConahay DR, Percutaneous Coronary Angioplasty with and without Prior Streptokinase Infusion for Treatment of Acute Myocardial Infarction, Am J Cardiol, 1982, 49, 1033.
5. Hartzler GO, Rutherford BD, McConahay DR, Johnson WL, Giorgi, LV, "High-Risk" Percutaneous Transluminal Coronary Angioplasty, Am J Cardiol 1988, 61, Suppl. G, 33G–37G.
6. Hartzler GO, Rutherford BD, McConahay DR, McCallister SH, Simultaneous Multiple Lesion Coronary Angioplasty – a Preferred Therapy for Patients with Multiple Vessel Disease, Circulation 982, 66, Suppl. II, II–5.
7. Kennedy JW, Kaiser GC, Fisher LD, Fritz JK, Myers W, Mudd JG, Ryan TJ Clinical and Angiographic Predictors of Operative Mortality from the Collaborative Study in Coronary Artery Surgery (CASS) Circulation 1981, 63, 793–802.
8. McCallister BD, Hartzler GO, Rutherford BD, McConahay DR, Palliative Percutaneous Transluminal Coronary Angioplasty for Unstable Angina in Patients, Circulation 1981, 64, Suppl. IV, IV–55.
9. McConahay DR, Hartzler GO, Rutherford BD, Percutaneous Transluminal Coronary Angioplasty: Use in Management of Symptomatic Patients with Recent Myocardial Infarction, Circulation 1982, 66, Suppl. II, II–329.
10. Mock MB, Holmes DR, Vlietstra RE, Gersh BJ, Detre KM, Kelsey SF, Orszulak TA, Schaff HV, Piehler JM, Van Raden MJ, Passamani ER, Kent KM, Gruentzig AR, Percutaneous Transluminal Coronary Angioplasty (PTCA) in the Elderly Patient: Experience in the National Heart, Lung, and Blood Institute PTCA Registry, Am J Cardiol, 1984, 53, Suppl. C, 89C–91C.

11. O'Keefe JH, Hartzler GO, Rutherford BD, McConahay DR, Johnson WL, Giorgi LV, Ligon RW, Left Main Coronary Angioplasty: Early and Late Results of 127 Acute and Elective Procedures, Am J Cardiol 1989, 64, 144-7.

Author's address:
Geoffrey O. Hartzler M.D.
c./o. Cardiovascular Consultants Inc.
Medical Plaza II-20
4320 Wornall Road
Kansas City, MO 64111, USA

Complications in New Interventional Techniques

Diagnostic Implications of Percutaneous Atherectomy: Angioscopic, Histologic, and Cell Culture Study

A. v. Pölnitz[1], G. Bauriedel[1], P. C. Dartsch[2], I. Schinko[3], D. Backa[1], E. Betz[2], U. Welsch[3] and B. Höfling[1]

[1]Ludwig-Maximilians-Universität München, Klinikium Großhadern, Medical Clinic I, Munich, FRG
[2]University of Tübingen, Institute of Physiology I, Tübingen, FRG
[3]Ludwig-Maximilians-Universität München, Anatomical Institute, Munich, FRG

Summary

In this study we report on percutaneous atherectomy, not only as a therapeutic modality, but also as a technique with diagnostic implications. The adjunctive use of angioscopy allows for the selective "biopsy" of plaque material, thus providing percutaneous access to the primary atherosclerotic process and to the phenomenon of restenosis. The Simpson atherectomy catheter was used to treat 40 patients with a total of 72 lesions of the iliac (n = 5), superficial femoral (n = 62), and popliteal (n = 5) arteries; five patients had rest pain and two had gangrene. The primary success rate was over 90%. The percent of stenosis decreased from 87.2 ± 14% to 16.6 ± 15.5%. In the longterm, angiographic restenosis was found in 21% of lesions with a difference seen based on primary morphology: 27% for concentrics, 5% for eccentrics, and 42% in total occlusions.

Angioscopic inspection of the treated segment was found to be helpful in identifying residual stenotic material or flaps, as well as in evaluating total occlusions, but it proved problematic for stenosis quantification. Light microscopy as well as electron microscopic study could identify smooth muscle cell proliferation and increased extracellular matrix as hallmarks of restenosis. Early cell culture studies show that growth of cell populations from atherectomy specimens are possible and that this model may prove to be a suitable method for the study of factors capable of inhibiting the restenosis process.

Percutaneous balloon angioplasty for the treatment of peripheral vascular disease is limited in the treatment of total occlusions and by the relatively high long-term restenosis rate of 20% to 45% [1–3]. Residual plaque material may contribute to this problem and therefore, new techniques which remove plaque material are being developed. The removal of plaque material, in addition to its therapeutic role, provides percutaneous access to the atherosclerotically altered vessel. Thus, histological and biochemical evaluation, as well as cell culture study of both primary lesions and restenoses are facilitated. We report on our results with the Simpson peripheral atherectomy catheter [4] which has been found to be safe and effective in peripheral vessels [5–7] and on the evaluation of removed atherectomy specimens with light phase [8] and electron microscopy [9], as well as results of initial cell culture studies [10].

Patients and methods

A total of 72 lesions in 40 patients with symptomatic peripheral vascular disease were treated with the atherectomy catheter. Five patients had rest pain and two had gangrene. The atherectomy procedure was performed under heparinization in the catheterization

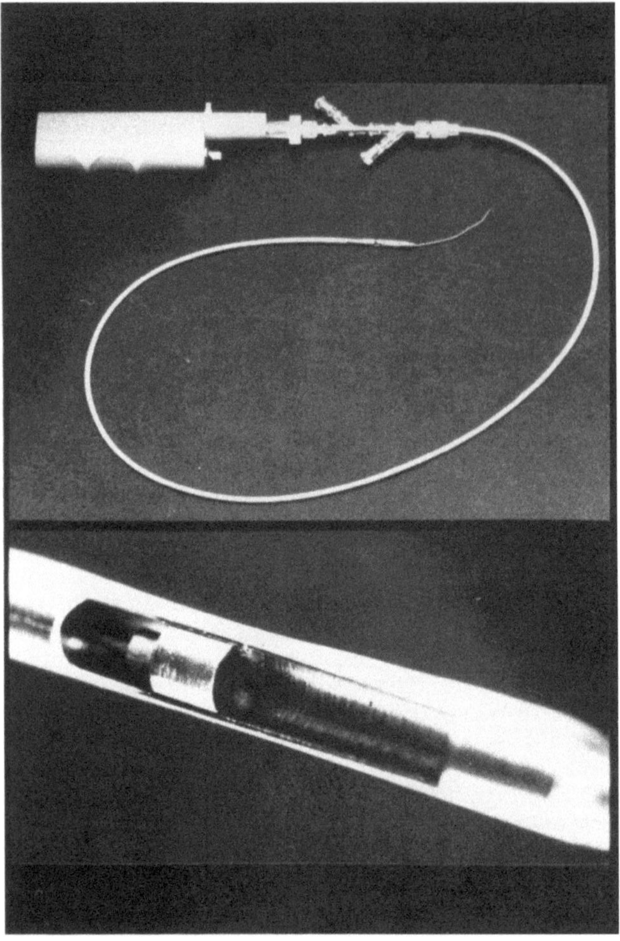

Fig. 1. The peripheral Simpson atherectomy catheter incorporates a guide wire at its tip, a cylindrical housing (enlargement), and a rotating cutting edge which is driven by a hand-controlled motor.

laboratory as previously described [5–7]. The essential feature of the catheter is a cylindrical housing with an opening encompassing one-third of its circumference at its tip (Fig. 1). Plaque material protruding into this opening can be excised and trapped in the distal housing cup. In the treatment of total occlusions a dotter technique using either a guide wire, catheter, or PTA is first necessary to establish a channel into which the atherectomy catheter can be placed. The lumen is then enlarged by the removal of plaque material.

Angioscopic evaluation was performed when feasible before, during, and after the intervention using a flexible fiberoptic endoscope (d = 1.5 or 1.0 mm, Miniflex Angioscope, American Edwards Lab.). If significant residual plaque material or flaps of the atherectomized segment were angioscopically detected and found to obstruct the recanalized lumen, they were localized by fluoroscopic control of thd position of the angioscope, and additional passes of the atherectomy catheter were performed prior to a final angioscopic inspection [11].

48

Histological evaluation (light-microscopy)

Excised specimens from 52 primary stenoses (iliac n = 5, superficial femoral artery n = 44, popliteal n = 3) of 24 patients (mean age 64.4 $\pm$ 8.8 years, 21 male, three female) were examined. Angiographically, the lesions were reduced from 84.4 $\pm$ 14.4% to 16.5 $\pm$ 12.5%. In addition, seven restenoses (angiographically > 50%) from five patients (all taking salicylates) occurring at a mean of 5.4 $\pm$ 2.5 months were re-atherectomized and histologically evaluated.

Transmission electron microscopy

A total of 55 tissue specimens from 14 patients undergoing atherectomy were analyzed with transmission electron microscopy. In this series the mean degree of stenosis was reduced from 95 $\pm$ 7% to 25 $\pm$ 11% (eight total occlusions and six high-grade stenoses of the femoral and popliteal arteries were treated). Immediately after percutaneous extraction, the plaque cylinders were fixed in 3.5% glutaraldehyde, postfixed in osmiumtetroxyd, dehydrated in a series of graded alcohol, and finally embedded in araldit. Ultrathin sections were stained with uranyl acetate and lead citrate and examined by a Zeiss EM 10 or a Phillips CM 10 electron microscope.

Cell culture study

Cell cultures of the excised atherectomy specimens were set using either an explant technique [11], or after enzymatic disaggregation using a modified technique [13]: briefly, the specimens were cut in 1 × 1 mm pieces and incubated for 180 min at 37°C in a collagenase/elastase solution. Separated cells were then centrifuged with 20% human serum, placed in cell culture, and bathed in Kollagen Type I. The culture medium used was a 1:1 mixture of Ham F12 and Waymouth's MB 752/1, with additional 15% pooled and heat-deactivated human serum and antibiotics. The cells were incubated at 37°C in a damp 7% carbon dioxide atmosphere.

Indirect immunofluorescence was performed using anti-smooth muscle cell alpha-actin (BioMakor) and anti-human factor VIII-related antigen (Ortho Diagnostic Systems).

Results are reported as mean $\pm$ SD. The paired Student's *t*-test (two-tailed) and chi-square tests were used to calculate significance of differences pre- and post-atherectomy. Significance was considered at the < 0.05 level.

Results

Angiographic results

Forty patients with 74 stenoses (iliac n = 5, superficial femoral n = 64, and popliteal n = 1) underwent atherectomy. Acute success (residual stenosis of < 50%) could be achieved in 91% of occlusions (19/21) and in 93% of stenoses (50/53). The mean (angiographic) stenosis was reduced from 87.2 $\pm$ 14% to 16.6 $\pm$ 15.5%.

A 6-month control angiography was performed in a total of 43 lesions. The mean 6-months stenosis was 35 $\pm$ 31%. Although not significant, there was a tendency for a higher mean 6-months-stenosis in the concentric (42.4%; n = 11) as compared to the eccentric lesions (25.7%; n = 20). Total occlusions showed the highest mean stenosis of 64.3%. An angiographic restenosis (defined as > 70%) was found in 9/43 lesions (21%).

300/88
191
IMAGE
115
MASK
15
- 97
HOEFLING/HUBER
KLIN. GROSSHADERN MED.I
23-FEB-88 / 12:46:32
PRAE   ATHEREKTOMIE

a

300/88
306
IMAGE
58
MASK
15
- 150
HOEFLING/HUBER
KLIN. GROSSHADERN MED.I
23-FEB-88 / 13:36:20
POST   ATHEREKTOMIE

b

50

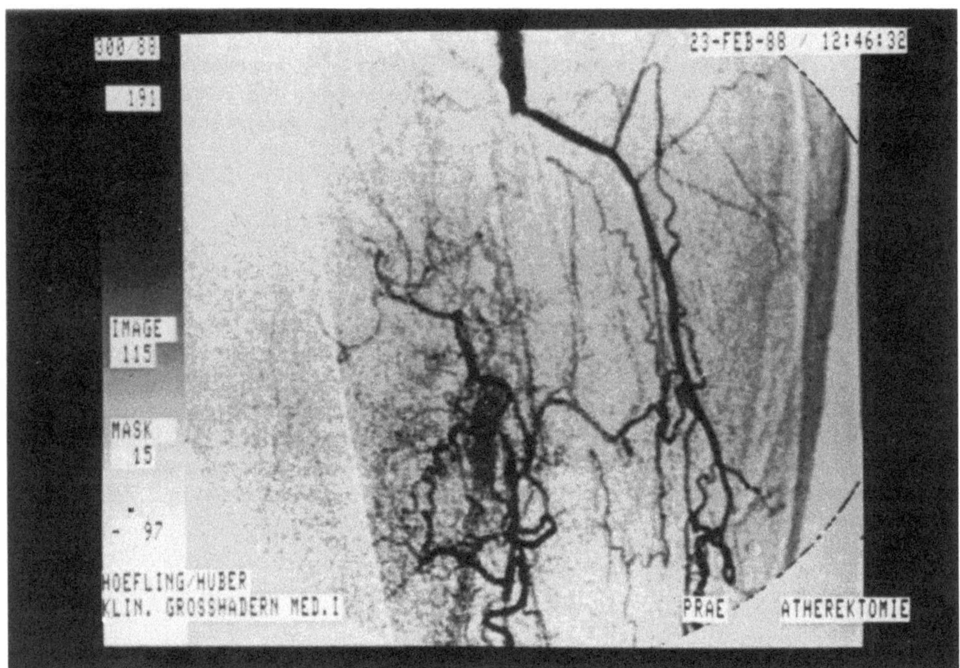

When analyzing for primary morphology a restenosis was found in 1/20 (5%) of eccentric lesions and in 3/11 (27%) of concentrics; total occlusions had a significantly higher restenosis rate of 42% (5/12).

Despite our efforts to optimize our results by angioscopic inspection of the treated site and the performance of additional passages of the atherectomy catheter should angioscopy detect residual stenoses or plaque material, there was no instance of vessel rupture or acute thrombosis. To date, there has been one incidence of clinically relevant distal embolization and two significant groin hematomas.

Angiographic examples

Figure 2 is of a total occlusion of the superficial femoral artery which was recanalized by an initial mechanical Dotter technique and then treated by atherectomy.

Angioscopic results

Angioscopic inspection of the superficial femoral or popliteal arteries was performed in 47 patients with a total of 62 lesions. Pre-atherectomy inspection usually revealed a red, pulsating vessel in the angiographically normal segments, while pale white or yellow plaque formation obstructing the lumen could be seen at the target lesion sites, qualitatively confirming the angiographic image. Occlusions could be clearly visualized with a total white-out of the image. In some cases, the occlusion could be crossed with the angioscope, and somewhat surprising was the finding of an occasional angiographic-long occlusion which, in actuality, was one or more shorter occlusions, with intermediated non-collateralized segments with a relatively intact vascular relief.

Qualitative angioscopic inspection was found to be a useful adjunct to the procedure in that residual obstructing flaps or plaques after atherectomy were occasionally not seen angiographically (Fig. 3). In addition, in cases of high grade stenosis (including 100% occlusions), initial passage of the angioscope or a guide wire under visual control may avoid guide wire- or catheter-induced complications.

Histological evaluation (light microscopy)

A mean of 5.9 $\pm$ 4.5 tissue specimens (max. 20, min. 1) were obtained per lesion. 305 specimens with a mean length of 4.9 $\pm$ 2.4 mm (max. 13 mm) and width of 1.3 $\pm$ 0.5 mm (max. 2 mm) were carefully examined. Macroscopically (Fig. 4) the specimens ranged from soft, white, and glistening tissue, sometimes with yellow streaks, to very yellow, fatty-appearing material.

Findings in primary stenoses

A total of 305 specimens from 52 stenoses were examined. A thickened intima was present in all stenoses, the internal elastic lamina in 42.3%, whereas media could be found in 55.8% of lesions. In addition, 75% of stenoses showed overlying thrombi. It is striking that endothelium was found in only 3.8%; this could be attributed to disruption of the cell

◄ **Fig. 2.** Total occlusion of the superficial femoral artery before (a) and after (b) mechanical recanalization and atherectomy.

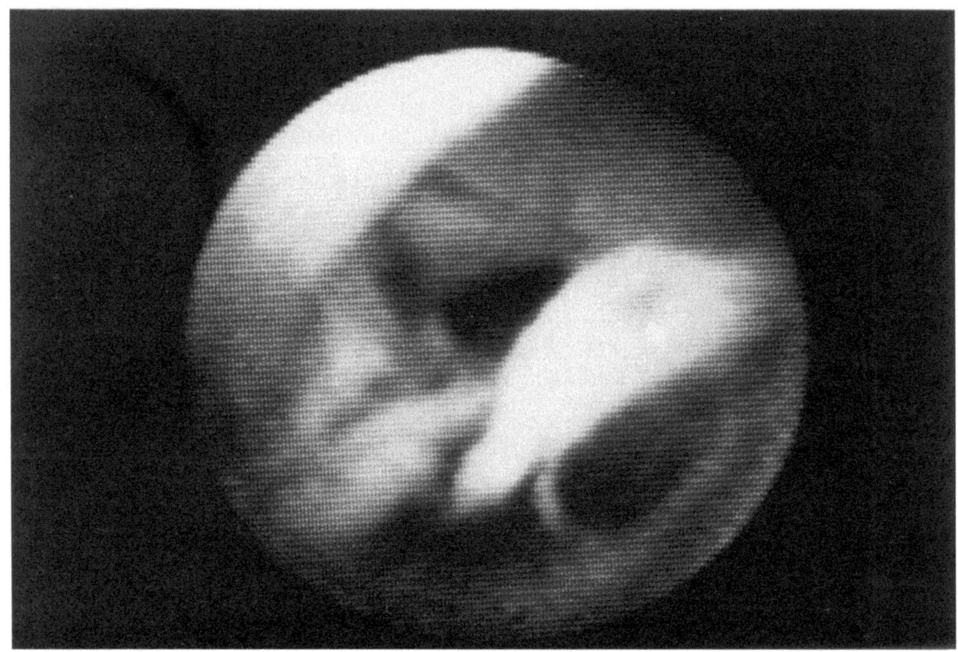

Fig. 3. Angioscopic view of a concentric lesion post-atherectomy. A large flap seen protruding into the vessel lumen could be subsequently removed with additional passes of the atherectomy catheter.

wall due to the atherectomy itself, or to the histological preparation process. It is important to note that neither the external elastic lamina nor the adventitia could be detected in any specimen. All intimal sections were thickened and showed regularly oriented smooth muscle-like (myointimal) cells surrounded by extracellular fibrotic matrix.

Findings in restenoses

All restenoses showed irregularly, non-longitudinally oriented cellular proliferation whose morphology ranged from a rather slender spindle shape to a more plump cell body with varying amounts of cytoplasm (Fig. 4). They were embedded within collagenous-like connective tissue. Furthermore, specimens from restenoses showed more foam cells and inflammatory infiltration. In addition, the media was reached in all restenotic lesions, and six of the seven had overlying organized thrombi.

In one patient atherectomy was performed for a restenosis 8 months after a primary angioplasty procedure. Histological evaluation in this instance showed that the major bulk of the excised specimens consisted of organized thrombus. In addition, the intima was thickened and fibrotic, and media was also present.

Electron microscopic results

Ultrastructurally, plaque material consisted of abundant extracellular matrix with collagen fibrils and elastic fibers or lamellae. Elongated and pancake-shaped smooth

52

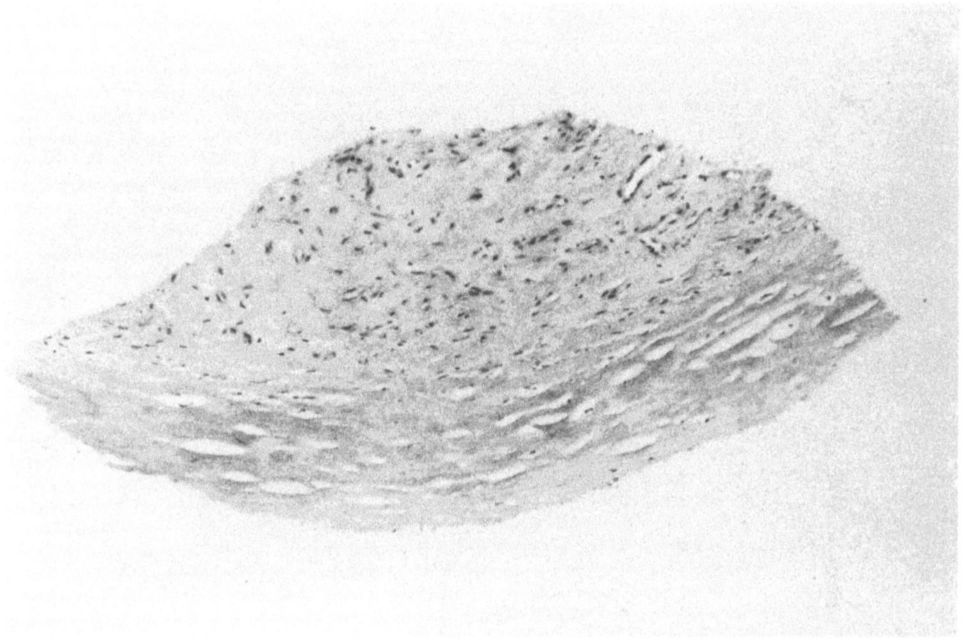

Fig. 4. Histological preparation of a specimen taken from a restenosis after atherectomy. Note the marked cellular proliferation overlying a thickened intima. This typical picture of myointimal proliferation was found in each restenosis evaluated. (Hematoxylin and Eosin, 10 ×).

muscle cells surrounded by an amorphous basal lamina of variable width were irregularly embedded in this matrix. Occasionally, thrombocytes, fibrin, and necrotic cells were found overlying the connective tissue. Endothelial cells were not observed.

In two patients, intra- and extracellular large cholesterol crystals could be detected. At the periphery, longitudinally oriented myofilament bundles were seen anchored in attachment plaques. Variable cell phenotypes were found, but cells particularly rich in filaments were not seen. The vast majority of the cells contained numerous cytoplasmic organelles, including perinuclear rough endoplasmic reticulum, Golgi complex, and mitrochondria as well as lysosomes (Fig. 5).

Cell culture studies

Initial studies showed that cell culture lines with predominantly elongated shaped smooth muscle cells, as characterized by anti-alpha actin immunofluorescence staining [14], could be grown from the plaque material removed with the atherectomy catheter [15]. The population doubling time of primary stenoses removed from 19 patients was found to be $0.16 \pm 0.04\%$ per day, while that of material removed after a restenosis was $0.64 \pm 0.15\%$ ($p < 0.001$) [15].

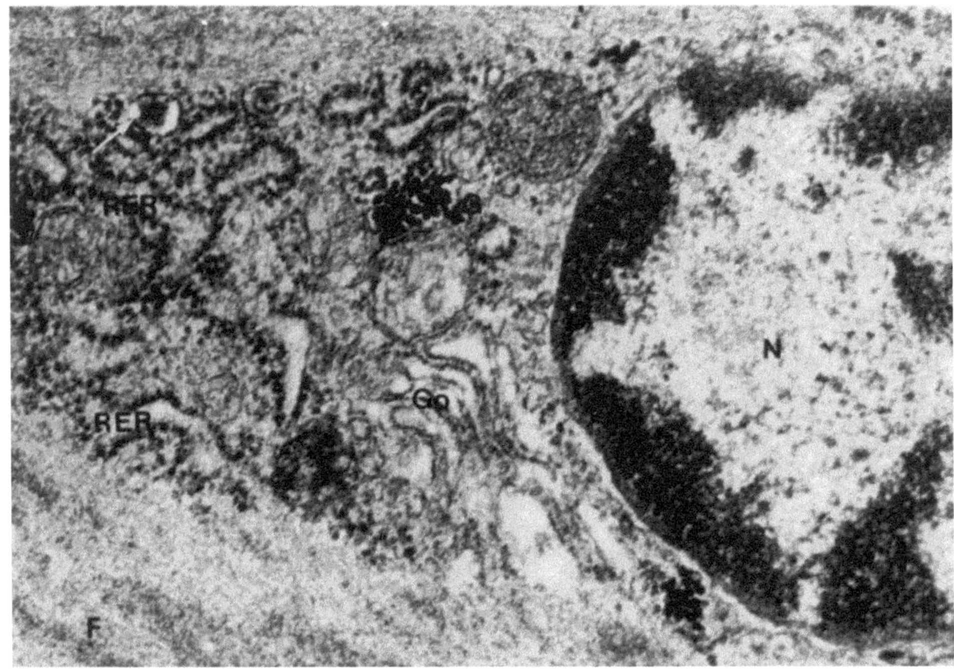

Fig. 5. Transmission electron microscopic view of a smooth muscle cell taken from atherectomized plaque material showing an increase in perinuclear rough endoplasmic reticulum (RER), Golgi complex (Go), and mitochondria, as well as lysosomes. (N: nucleus; × 48000).

Discussion

The ability of the catheter to smoothly remove plaque material is important in that a) it perhaps lowers the long-term restenosis rate; b) the risk of distal embolization is largely eliminated; and c) the biopsy of plaque material, especially under angioscopic guidance, for histologic, biochemical, and cell culture study may provide useful models for studying the process of restenosis and its pharmacological prevention.

Classical light phase histological studies showed that, although atherosclerotic plaque material was also obtained, the classic atheromatous bed was only rarely present. It was rather a thickened, fibrotic intima with or without thrombus overlying the actual plaque that was mainly removed by atherectomy. Evaluation of seven restenoses compared with their primary lesions showed more irregular fibrocellular proliferation and inflammatory infiltrates. In addition, some degree of organized thrombus was found in the majority (6/7) of restenoses.

The presence of smooth muscle cell proliferation in atherosclerotic material, both primarily and after balloon injury has been previously well described [16–19]. Smooth muscle cells migrating into the intima have been shown to exhibit a synthetic phenotype, with increased synthetic organelles, loss of the capacity to contract, and increased capacity to divide [20] and synthesize large amounts of extracellular matrix [21]. The electron microscope of our atherectomy specimens of primary stenoses characterized the smooth muscle cells as those of the intermediate phenotype surrounded by extensive extracellular matrix.

A higher doubling time of the smooth muscle cells of restenotic lesions as compared to primary lesions after atherectomy were found in culture, also suggesting an increased metabolic activity. Further study of such specimens will be useful in the characterization of growth characteristics and metabolic alterations of plaque smooth muscle cells. The signals for smooth muscle cell migration and proliferation may include PDGF, mitogenic factors released from dead smooth muscle cells, and endothelial and macrophage-derived growth factors; however, in-vivo evidence is still lacking.

Many substances are currently being evaluated for use after an interventional procedure in an effort to limit the process of restenosis: monoclonal antibodies to platelet receptors, prostaglandin E1, low molecular weight heparin, thromboxane synthetase inhibitors, hirudin, platelet-cAMP inhibitors and sulfinpyrazone, as well as calcium antagonists. Their additional evaluation in a cell culture model grown from atherectomy specimens could be advantageous; however, whether in vitro effects can be translated to in vivo activity remain to be tested.

References

1. Zeitler E, Richter EI, Seyferth W (1982) Femoropopliteal arteries. In: Percutaneous Transluminal Angioplasty. Dotter CT, Gruntzig AR, Shoop W (eds): Percutaneous Transluminal Angioplasty, New York, Springer Verlag, p. 105
2. Schneider E, Gruntzig A, Bollinger A (1982) Langzeitergebnisse nach perkutaner transluminaler Angioplastie (PTA) bei 882 konsekutiven Patienten mit iliacalen und femoro-poplitealen Obstruktionen. VASA 11: 322
3. Krepel VM, van Andel GJ, van Erp, Breslau PJ (1985) Percutaneous transluminal angioplasty of the femoropopliteal artery: Initial and long-term results. Radiology 156: 325
4. Simpson JB, Johnson DE, Thapliyal HV et al. (1985) Transluminal atherectomy: A new approach to the treatment of atherosclerotic vascular disease. Circulation 72, Supp II, III-146 (abst)
5. Simpson JB, Selmon MR, Robertson GC et al. (1988) Transluminal atherectomy for occlusive peripheral vascular disease. Am J Cardiol 61: 14: 96G–101G
6. Höfling B, von Pölnitz A, Backa D et al. (1988) Percutaneous removal of atheromatous plaques in peripheral arteries. Lancet I: 384–387
7. Höfling B, von Pölnitz A, Backa D et al. (1989) Angiographische und funktionelle Ergebnisse sowie histologische Befunde nach perkutaner Atherektomie bei Patienten mit arterieller Verschlußkrankheit. Z Kardiol 75 (in press)
8. von Pölnitz A, Backa D, Nerlich A, Höfling B (1989) Histological evaluation of "vessel-biopsies" obtained with the Simpson atherectomy catheter. J Am Coll Cardiol 13: 2: 149A
9. Schinko I, Bauriedel G, Höfling B, Welsch U (1989) Ultrastrukturelle und histochemische Befunde an Plaqumaterial, das mit dem Simpson-Atherektomiekatherter extrahiert wurde. In Assman G (ed): Arteriosklerose, neue Aspekte aus Zellbiologie und Molekulargenetik, Epidemologie und Klinik. Zuckschwerdt, München (in press)
10. Bauridel G, Dartsch PC, Voisard R, et al. (1989) Selective percutaneous biopsy of atheromatous plaque tissue for cell culture. Basic Res Cardiol (in press)
11. Höfling B, von Pölnitz A, Baurtiedel G et al. (1989) Use of Angioscopy to assess the results of percutaneous atherectomy. American Journal of Cardiac Imaging. 3: 20–26.
12. Chamley-Campbell JH, Campbell GR, Ross R (1979) The smooth muscle cell in culture. Phys Rev 59: 1.
13. Dartsch PC, Hämmerle H (1986) Orientation response of arterial smooth muscle cells to mechanical stimulation. Eur J Cell Biol 41: 339
14. Skalli O, Ropraz P, Trzeciak A et al. (1986) A monoclonal antibody against alpha-smooth muscle actin: A new probe for smooth muscle differentiation. J Cell Biol 103: 2787–2796
15. Dartsch PC, Bauriedel G, Höfling B, Betz E (1989) Cewll culture of human atheromatous plaque material. In Interventional Cardiology and Angiology. Höfling B and Pölnitz Av (eds). Steinkopff Verlag, Darmstadt, FRG. p. 119–129
16. Ross R, Glomset JA (1976) The pathogenesis of atherosclerosis (Part I). New Engl J Med 295: 369–377

17. Ross R, Glomset JA (1976) The pathogenesis of atherosclerosis (Part II). New Engl J Med 295: 420–425
18. Schwartz SM, Campbell GR, Campbell JH (1986) Replication of smooth muscle cells in vascular disease. Circ Res 58: 427–444
19. Waller BF (1987) Pathology of transluminal balloon angioplasty used in the treatment of coronary disease. Hum Pathol 18(5): 476–484
20. Ohara T, Nanto S, Asada S et al. (1988) Ultra-structural study of proliferating and migrating smooth muscle cells at the site of PTCA as an explanation for restenosis (abstract) Circulation 78: Suppl II: II–290
21. Campbell JH, Campbell GR (1987) Chemical stimuli of the hypertrophic response to smooth muscle, in Seidel CL (ed): Hypertrophic Response of Smooth Muscle. Boca Raton, Fla, CRC Press, pp 153–192

Author's address:
Dr A.v. Pölnitz
Klinikum Großhadern
Medizinische Klinik I
Marchioninistr. 15
8000 München 70, FRG

High-Frequency Rotational Angioplasty

R. Erbel, M. Haude, S. Iversen[1], U. Nixdorff, H. Oelert[1], U. Dietz and J. Meyer

II. Medical Clinic, Johannes Gutenberg-University Mainz, FRG
Department of Thoracic and Cardiovascular Surgery[1]

High frequency rotational angioplasty of coronary artery disease

In 19 patients with significant coronary artery disease, PTCR was used instead of PTCA. The PTCR was successful in all patients, but in nine patients additional PTCA was successfully performed. Coronary luminal narrowing could be reduced from 78 $\pm$ 19% to 32 $\pm$ 14% after rotablation and by combined treatment to 21 $\pm$ 14%. Only in one patient did coronary dissection occur; the patient was sent to surgery and had an uneventful outcome. No vessel perforation was observed. In one patient peripheral diagonal branch occlusion occurred. All vessels were open according to 24-control coronary angiography. Restenosis (> 70% stenosis) occurred in 4/15 patients controlled after 6 months, mainly in those with vessel occlusion (3/4).

PTCR seems to be a promising new technique. The indication for PTCR seems to be hard and long lesions which cannot be passed with the balloon. Possibly, the restenosis rate can be reduced.

Introduction

Percutaneous transluminal coronary angioplasty has become an important therapeutic method for treatment of patients with stable and unstable angina pectoris [19, 26, 27, 29]. The success rate of PTCA is > 90% [26, 35]; in patients with chronic occlusion it is between 45–71% [10, 21, 31]. The restenosis rate in patients with stable angina pectoris is between 20–30%, but in patients with unstable angina it is between 30–45% [27], and after recanalization it is 50% [10, 21, 31]. In order to increase the success rate in reopening of occluded vessels and to reduce the restenosis rate, high frequency [4, 25, 28] and low frequency [36, 37] rotational angioplasty devices were developed. These methods are alternatives to the laser systems [1, 3, 4, 6, 15].

In our report the use of the high frequency rotational angioplasty systems developed by David Auth Bellevue, Washington is described.

Methods

After diagnostic heart catheterization, indication for angioplasty was found in 19 patients. Premedication was used according to previous reports [26, 27, 29]. Patients received 20 ml Promit as Hapten and 100 ml/h low molecular dextran (Rheomacrodex) started 2–3 h before rotablation. 500 mg acetylsalicylic acid (Colfarit) was given the day before and the morning of the treatment. After intravenous puncture and advance of Swan Ganz catheter 10 000 IE heparine were injected. During the heart catheterization the patients received 3 mg/h nitroglycerine (Perlinganit) and 0.5 mg nifedipine (Adalat) for avoiding coronary spasm [12].

For rotablation the high frequency rotating angioplasty device of Auth [2, 11, 12, 14,

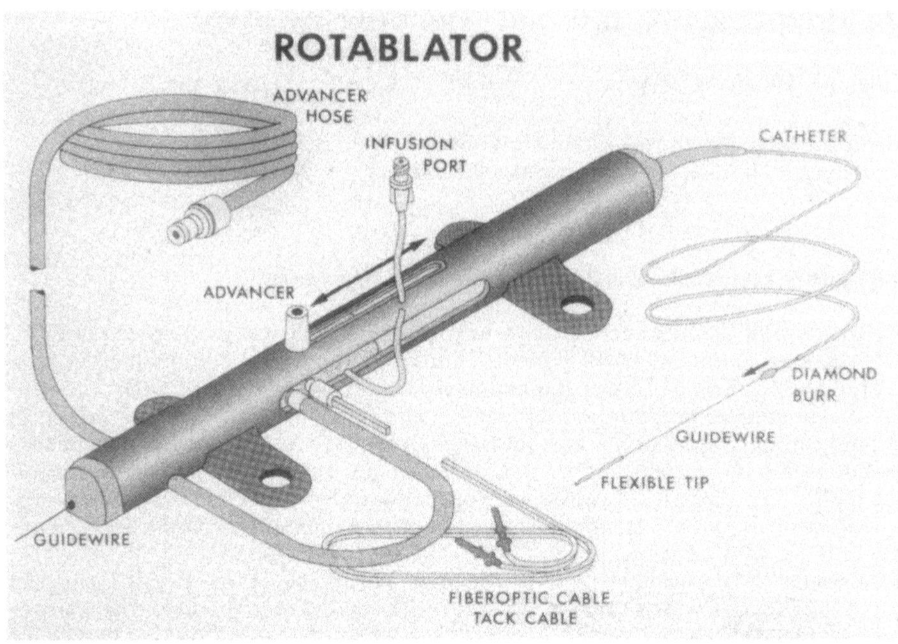

Fig. 1. Schematic drawing of the rotablation system with the infusion board, advancer catheter, guide wire and fiberoptic cable [12].

28] was used (Fig. 1). The stainless steel burr was coated with 30–80 μm diameter diamonds connected to a flexible catheter system that could be advanced over a central guide (0.009 inch) with a 2.5-cm long stainless steel spring tip. The drive shaft was connected to a compressed air driven motor. The guide wire was attached to a handle which allowed the operator to extend the wire tip or to rotate the guide wire in all down coronary artery branches. The turbine rotates the drive shaft at 150–190,000 rpm. A fiberoptic light probe measured the number of revolutions/min, which was displayed on the control panel. The speed could be controlled by a dial on the control panel and by a separate foot pedal that turns the turbine on or off. The turbine also pumps sterile saline solution into the plastic sheath to lubricate the rotating drive shaft and burr. By moving the control knob on the top of the plastic focus the operator could advance the burr along the guide wire. The burr travels at a speed of approximately 0.25 mm/s as its tip grades millions of microscopic particles, 90% of which are smaller than 10 μm [2, 28]. The entire system is sterile and used one time only (Biophysics, Bellevue, Washington, USA) [12]. Burrs of sizes between 1.25 mm and 2.25 mm for coronary arteries are available. The length of the catheters are 95 or 135 cm and guide wires are 270 cm. In patients where the positioning of the steel wire is difficult, first a recanalization catheter 3F (Schneider) was used for guiding the stainless steel wire of the rotablator as an exchange wire. After advancing of the burr into the coronary artery the position of the burr was controlled by contrast injection in order to avoid rotablation of healthy branches of the artery. During rotablation the speed is carefully controlled in order to avoid lowering the rotation speed by more than 10–20% of the starting speed. The rotation periods were between 5–10 s. The periods were short in order to avoid ischemic periods and in order to induce only a short period of ablation of plaque material. After the passage of the coronary luminal narrowing the burr was

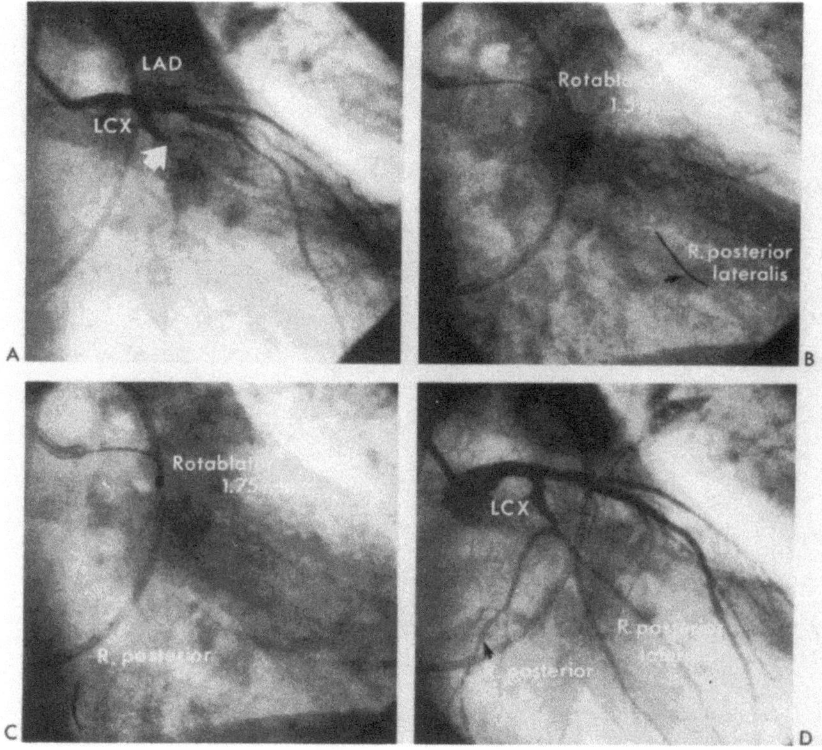

Fig. 2. Left coronary artery showing occlusion of the circumflex branch. A: before advancing the 1.5 mm burr; B: while advancing the 1.5 mm burr; C: rotational angioplasty with 1.75 mm burr; D: control coronary angiography [11].

advanced two or three times. The control coronary angiogram was repeated after intra-coronary injection of 0.2 mg nitroglycerine and 3,000 IE heparine.

Patients were sent to the intensive care unit after the procedure and received 15–17 IE heparine/kg/h and 3 mg/h nitroglycerine intravenously. After 24 h control ventriculogram and coronarograms in identical positions were performed. Follow-up treatment was identical to PTCA treatment and included 500 mg acetylsalicylic acid (Colfarit) and 3 × 10–20 mg nifedipine (Adalat) tid.

Patients had given their informed consent.

For calculation of left ventricular volume a disc method was used and ejection fraction was calculated. Coronary angiograms were evaluated by a partially automatic computer system and area stenosis were measured. (12)

All values are given as single and biplane values. P value below 0.5 was judged as 0.5.

Results

Rotation ablation was performed in 19 patients with significant stenosis of the left anterior descending coronary artery (n = 9) and of the right coronary artery (n = 5) and occluded vessels (n = 5) of the circumflex coronary artery (n = 3) and left descending coronary artery (n = 2).

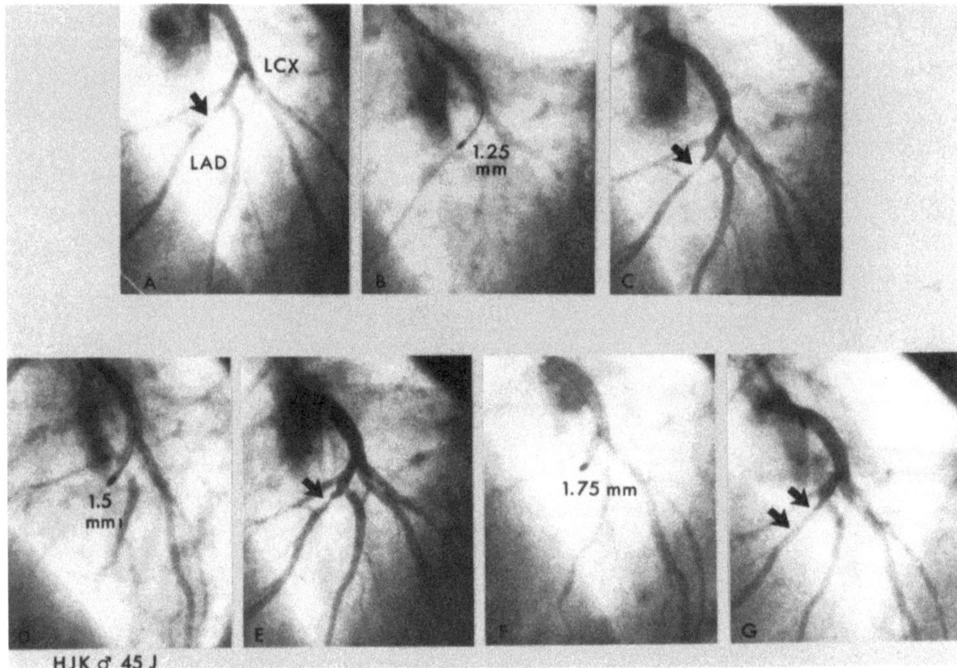

Fig. 3. Left coronary angiogram with high-grade lesion of the left anterior descending coronary artery (LAD) with normal left circumflex coronary artery (LCx). (A) Advancing of the 1.25 mm, 1.5 mm, and 1.75 mm burrs (B, D, F) are demonstrated, as well as the control angiograms (C, E, G). Coronary luminal narrowing is reduced and a vessel with smooth surface is visible.

A typical example of rotation ablation of an occluded circumflex coronary artery is given in Fig. 2 demonstrating that, even in angled coronary arteries, successful rotablation can be performed.

In Fig. 1 the rotablation of the left anterior descending coronary artery with different burr size is demonstrated. A smooth vessel surface was created. Also in the right coronary artery smooth surfaces could be formed with rotation ablation. Even an occlusion of the left anterior descending coronary artery could be recanalized as demonstrated in Fig. 5. In this patient a residual luminal narrowing PTCA was performed with a successful result.

Rotation ablation was successful in 18/19 patients, but additional PTCA was performed in 9/19 patients as a result of residual luminal narrowing. Coronary stenoses were reduced from 78 ± 19% to 32 ± 14%, and further to 21 ± 14% after rotation ablation and additional PTCA.

Usually the patient felt nothing during the rotational procedure and no pain occurred. In some patients chest discomfort developed apart from angina pectoris. This chest discomfort, described as a compression, was relieved during the next few hours. In one patient after rotation ablation of a coronary stenosis and reopening of two branches of the circumflex coronary artery (Fig. 6) severe chest pain developed on the intensive care unit. In the ECG, ST-segment elevation was evident and echocardiography revealed a localized pericardial effusion near the postero-lateral wall. Control coronary angiography revealed an open coronary vessel. In one patient after rotation ablation of a proximal high-grade coronary lesion with a 1.5 mm burr only a small increase of luminal diameter could be

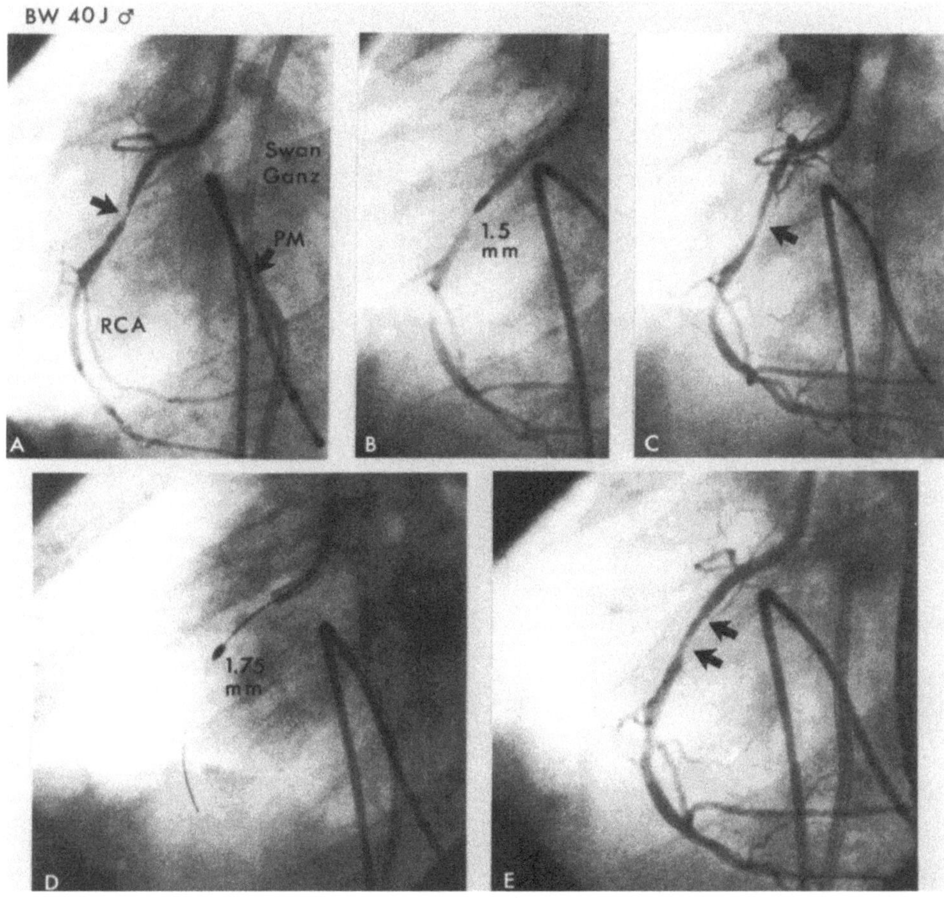

Fig. 4. Right coronary angiogram before (A) and after (C, E) rotablation with a 1.5 mm burr (B) and 1.75 mm burr (D). Reduction of coronary luminal narrowing and a vessel with smooth surface [12].

demonstrated (Fig. 7). Therefore, a 2.0 mm burr was used. During the rotation ablation a drop in the speed to 146,000 rpm occurred. Control coronary angiogram demonstrated a very rough surface of the left anterior descending coronary artery and flaps as signs of coronary dissection. After immediate bypass surgery the patient could be discharged.

In one patient (Fig. 8) a side branch of the diagonal branch of the left anterior descending coronary artery occluded after recanalization of the left anterior descending coronary artery (Fig. 5). During follow-up a CK elevation up to 150 U/l developed due to the side branch occlusion (Fig. 8). Control cineventriculography demonstrated wall motion abnormality in the mid part of the anterior wall (Fig. 9) which resolved during follow-up. The 6-month control angiogram was normal (Fig. 9).

In order to detect embolization-induced ischemia control ventriculograms after 24 h were analyzed. No significant changes of systolic volume or ejection fraction occurred and segmental wall motion was unchanged. Only in the patient with the embolism (Fig. 9) segmental wall motion abnormalities were seen.

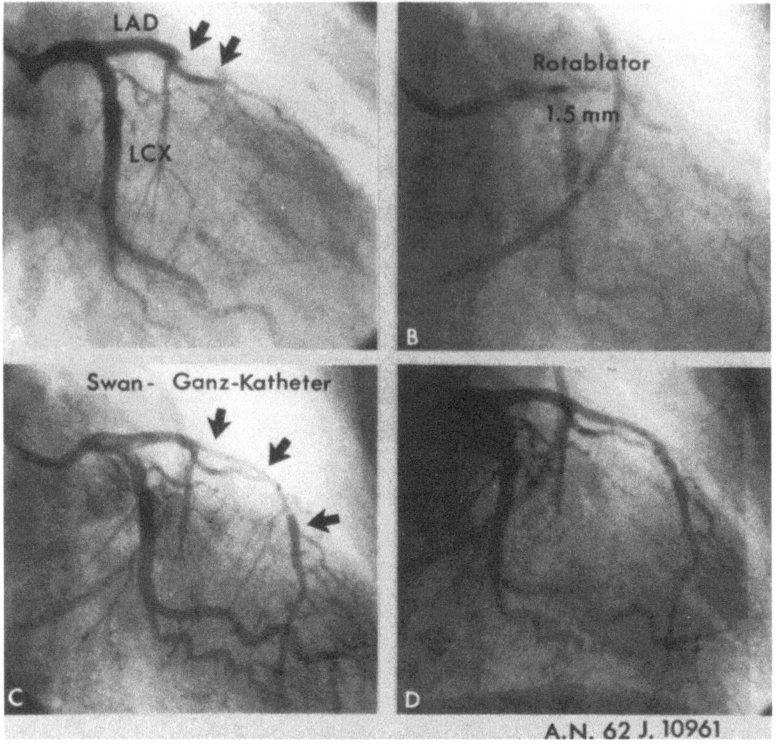

Fig. 5. Left coronary angiogram in a patient before and after reopening of an occluded left anterior descending coronary artery (LAD) with a 1.5 mm burr (B). The result after rotation ablation demonstrated residual luminal narrowing (C) which was reduced with additional balloon angioplasty resulting in a free and open vessel with smooth surface (D).

Complete thallium-201 studies (n = 7) before and after rotation demonstrated improved uptake and no ablation signs of new thallium-201 defects.

The 6-month control showed restenosis in 3/5 recanalized vessels, in 1/5 patients with rotation ablation alone, but in no patient (n = 5) with additional PTCA.

Discussion

Angioplasty of stable and unstable angina is still the method of choice in single-vessel disease and has a success rate of 90% [27, 29, 30, 32]. The restenosis rate is between 20–30% and is not influenced by acetylsalicylic-acid [30], calcium-antagonists [38] or molsidomin [7]. In 1–7%, emergency bypass surgery is necessary [32].

In order to increase the success rate in occluded vessels and to reduce restenosis rate, but also in order to treat longer lesions, mechanical systems were developed. We could demonstrate that coronary arteries can be reopened and luminal narrowing reduced by rotation ablation [8, 11, 12]. The systems can be used not only in the proximal, but also in peripheral parts of the artery.

It is an advantage that usually the patient does not feel the procedure itself. Ischemic

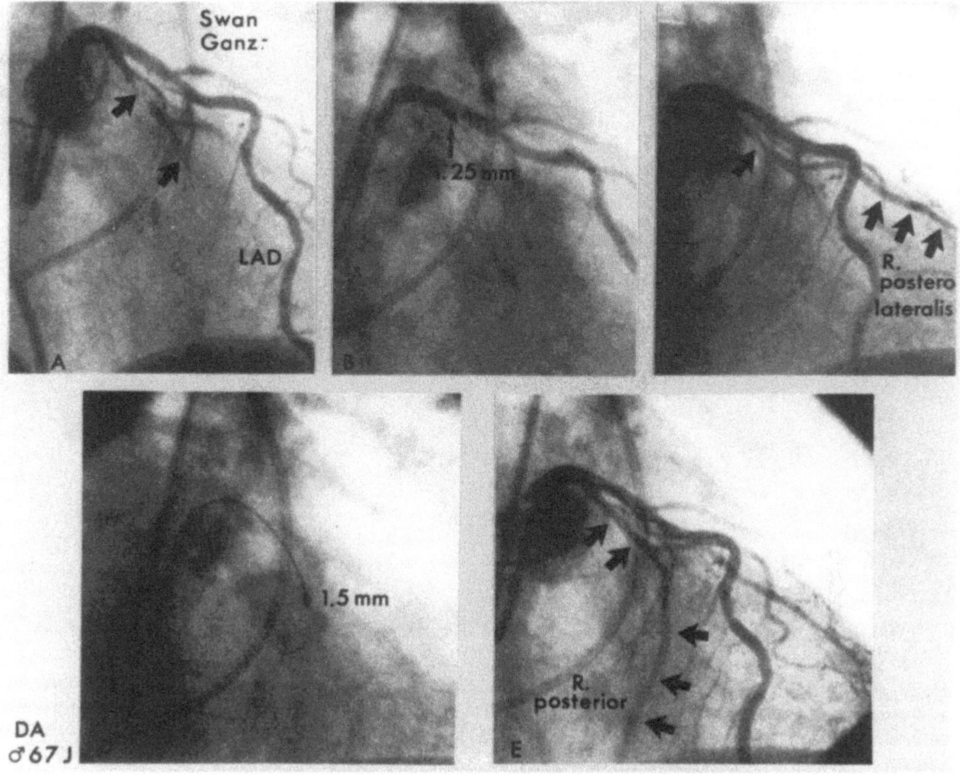

Fig. 6. Left coronary angiogram in a patient with a proximal stenosis and a distal occlusion of the left circumflex coronary artery. The stenosis was reduced and the vessel occlusion of the postero-lateral and the posterior branch of the left circumflex coronary artery (RCx) was recanalized.

periods such as during PTCA were not observed, possibly due to the short rotation periods of 5–10 s.

The rotablator has the advantage that there is no electric contact between the patient and the driver system, as there is with other rotation devices [25]. The speed is controlled with fiberoptic connection. It is also an advantage that the usual pressurized air of the catheterization laboratory can be used. The system is well constructed and easy to handle.

As an alternative to the rotation ablation, low-frequency rotational angioplasty devices using wires with burrs were developed; they use speeds of 100–200 rpm. Experimental [36] and clinical studies [37] have shown that occlusions can be opened without perforation. Whereas additional PTCA is used with low frequency system, rotation ablation can reduce coronary luminal narrowing step-by-step using increasing sizes of the burr. Additional examinations in larger patient collectives will demonstrate if the different results after rotation ablation are related to the structure of the stenosis. It seems to be the case that in sclerotic lesions the success rate is much better than in excentric or soft lesions [12, 13].

The Simpson catheter is able to cut parts of the coronary artery and to remove these parts [33]. Thermal processes are used with radio frequency angioplasty in order to open reocclusions and reduce restenosis [16, 17]. These effects are also used for laser angioplasty [3, 4–6, 14, 20]. First results with laser coronary angioplasty and peripheral coronary

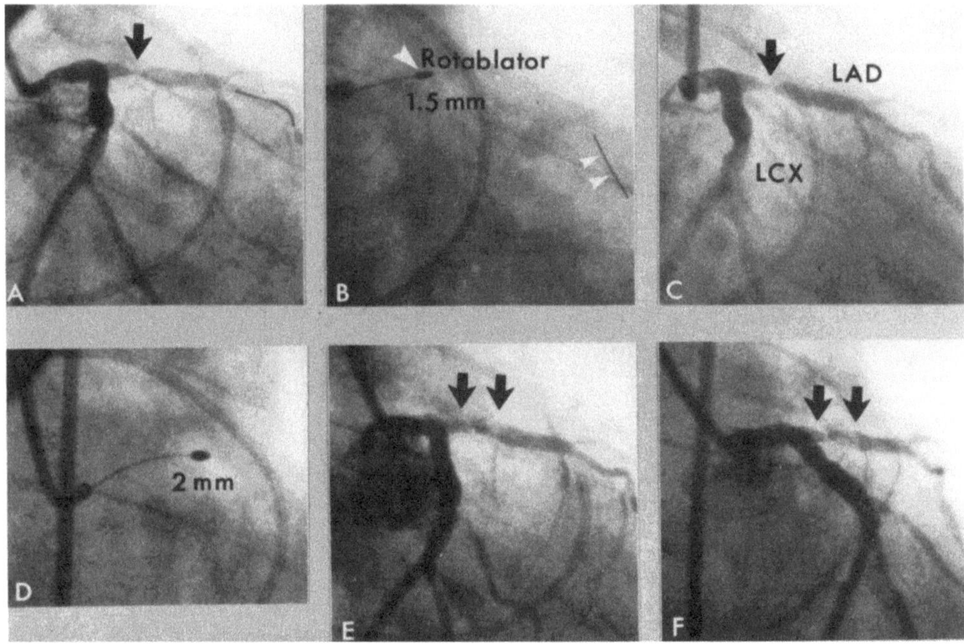

Fig. 7. Left coronary angiogram with demonstration of a high-grade proximal coronary stenosis before (A) and after treatment with a 1.5 mm burr (B). After use of a 2 mm burr (D) flow reduction, rough coronary surface, and filling defects as a result of vessel dissection (E, F). Patient underwent successful bypass surgery.

angioplasty have been published [4–6]. With the use of mechanical as well as thermal devices peripheral embolism can occur [2–6, 15, 17, 20, 22, 33, 34, 44]. The analysis of ventricular volumes and wall motion in our patients demonstrated that a diffuse myocardial ischemia during the rotation ablation is not induced. Only in the patient with the side branch occlusion did a CK elevation up to 150 U/l occur.

Perforations can occur with all mechanical and thermal devices [2]. It cannot be excluded that the observed pericarditis is a beginning penetration of the vessel with inflammatory infiltration of the pericardium. The perforation danger is much higher with laser techniques [1, 4]. With PTCA, perforations are rare but they can occur [18] and are experimentally observed also with radio frequency angioplasty [17].

The mechanism of balloon angioplasty is the induction of intima and media dissection [9]. Histological examinations after high-frequency rotational angioplasty also demonstrated that intima and media dissection can occur but were not the usual mechanism in the method [2, 28]. In our group of patients dissection of the vessel was observed in one patient who was sent immediately to surgery. That means that, even for rotation ablation, an anesthesiologist and cardiac surgery team must be available.

Early thrombotic occlusions were not observed under treatment with acetylsalicylic acid under full heparinization. This is important, because using the rotablator over a length of 2–3 cm the coronary artery is treated and thus, a large part of the vessel is open to platelet adhesion and the vessel endothelian is nearly denuded. In comparison to PTCA, the length of the vessel treated by rotation ablation is identical.

The restenosis rate seems to be not enhanced. The early results demonstrate a possible

64

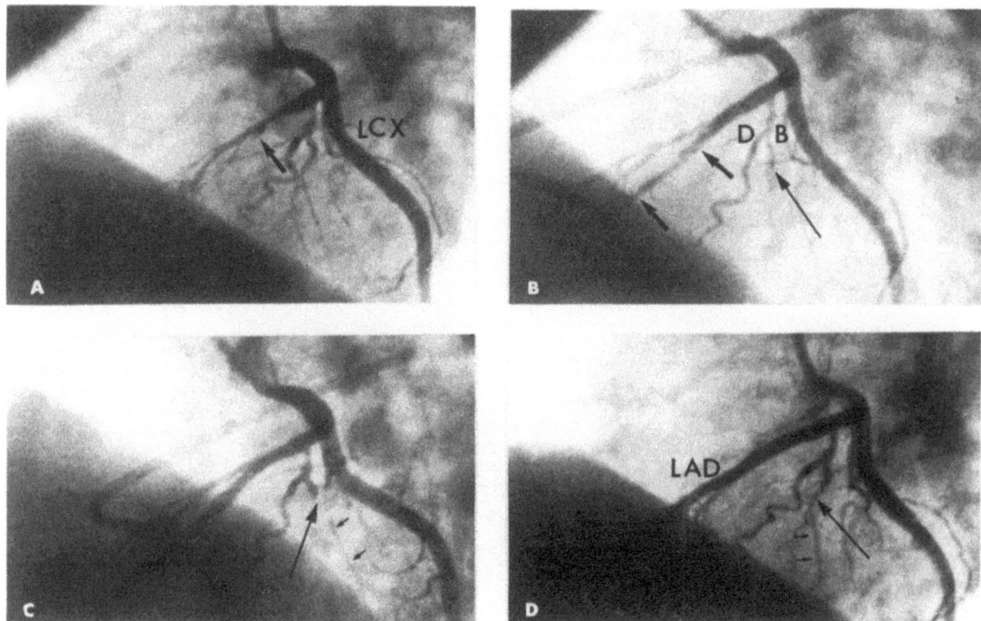

Fig. 8. Left coronary angiogram in the LAO projection in a patient with occluded left anterior descending coronary artery (a). After reopening of LAD by rotablation (b), occlusion of a side branch (B) of the diagonal branch (D) of the LAD is observed (c). Persistent occlusion is demonstrated after 24 h with reopening after 6 months (d).

reduction of restenosis rate. Only one restenosis in 10 patients with stenosis was observed. The restenosis and occlusion occurred mainly in patients with recanalized coronary vessels.

Clinical implication

Rotablation seems to be a promising new technique for opening occluded vessels and for reduction of coronary luminal narrowing. Success rate seems to be related to the degree of rigidity of the stenosis. If restenosis rate can be reduced, rotablation will become an alternative method to PTCA and is an additional method in patients in whom balloons can not pass the lesion.

Acknowledgement: We thank all technicians and nurses of the catheterization laboratory, Miss M. Meurer for her graphic, and Mrs. Herbrik for her secretarial work. We thank Biophysics, particularly Miss Louise Myers, for her support.

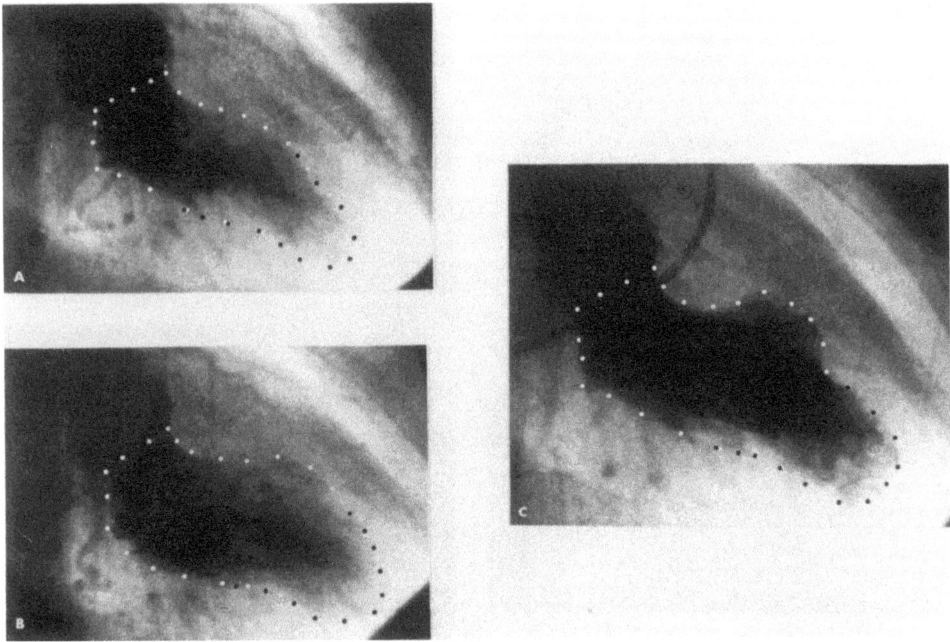

Fig. 9. Cineventriculogram of the patient in Fig. 8 before (a), immediately after rotablation (b) and 6 months later (c), showing that side branch occlusion induced segmental wall motion abnormalities which resolved during follow-up.

References

1. Abela GS, Norman SK, Cohen DM, Franzini D, Feldman RL, Crea F, Fenech A, Pepine CJ, Conti CR (1985) Laser recanalization of occluded artherosclerotic arteries in vivo and in vitro. Circulation 71: 403
2. Ahn SS, Auth D, Marcus DR, Moore WS (1988) Removal of focal atheromatous lesions by angioscopically guided high-speed rotary atherectomy. J Vasc Surg 7: 292
3. Biamino G, Harnoss BM, Kar H, Dörschel K, Müller G (1988) Experience in excimer laser photoablation of arterio-sclerotic plaques. In: Advances in Laser Medicine I, ecomed, Landsberg 147
4. Crea F, Davies G, McKenna WJ, Pashazadeh M, Keogh B, Kidner P, Taylor KM, Maseri A (1988) Percutaneous coronary laser recanalisation with metal-capped optical fibres in man. In: Advances in Laser Medicine I, ecomed, Landsberg 227
5. Cumberland DC, Tayler DI, Welsh CL, Guben JK, Sanborn TA, Moore DJ, Greenfield AJ, Ryan TJ (1986) Results with a laser probe in total peripheral artery occlusions. Lancet 1457
6. Cumberland DC, Oakley GDG, Smith GH, Tayler DI, Starkey IR, Fleming JS, Goiti JJ, Davis J (1986) Percutaneous laser-assisted coronary angioplasty. Lancet 214
7. Darius H, Erbel R, Schmucker B, Reusch U, Meyer J (1988) Effets anti-ischémique du SIN-1, métabolite de la mosidomine, au cours de l'angioplastie coronarienne et effets antiplaquettaires chez l'homme. Presse Méd 17: 1033
8. Dietz U, Erbel R, Haude M, Nixdorff U, Iversen S, Pannen P, Meyer J (1989) Angiographische und histologische Befunde bei der koronaren Hochfrequenz-Rotationsatherektomie in vitro. Z Kardiol 78, Suppl 1–104
9. Düber C, Jungbluth A, Rumpelt HJ, Erbel R, Meyer J, Thoenes W (1986) Morphology of the coronary arteries after combined thrombolysis and percutaneous transluminal coronary angioplasty for acute myocardial infarction. Am J Cardiol 58: 698

10. Erbel R, Diefenbach C, Schriber G, Pop T, Vorshausen K, Rupprecht HZ, Aydin A, Meyer J (1986) Retardization of totally occluded coronary vessels by percutaneous trans-luminal coronary angioplasty. In: Höffling B (ed) Current problems in PTCA. Steinkopf Darnstadt pp 109

11. Erbel R, O'Neill W, Auth D, Haude M, Nixdorff U, Rupprecht HJ, Dietz U, Meyer J (1989) High-frequency rotablation of occluded coronary artery during heart catheterization. Cath Cardiovasc Diagn 17: 56

12. Erbel R, O'Neill W, Auth D, Haude M, Nixdorff U, Dietz U, Rupprecht HJ, Tschollar W, Meyer J (1989) Hochfrequenz-Rotationsatherektomie bei koronarer Herzkrankheit. Dtsch Med Wochenschr 114: 487

13. Fourrier JL, Auth D, Lablanche JM, Brunetaud JM, Gommeaux A, Bertrand ME (1988) First percutaneous coronary rotational atherectomies in man. Eur Heart J 9, Suppl 1: 336

14. Hansen DD, Auth DC, Vracko R, Ritchie JL (1988) Rotational atherectomy in atherosclerotic rabbit iliac arteries. Am Heart J 115: 160

15. Heintzen MP, Neubaur T, Klepzig M, Richter EI, Zeitler E, Strauer BE (1988) Clinical Experiences in Nd: YAG laser angioplasty in the periphery. In: Advances in Laser Medicine I, ecomed, Landsberg 103

16. Höher M, Hombach V, Höpp HW, Eggeling T, Kochs M, Hilger HH (1988) Intrakoronare Hochfrequenzangioplastie: erste klinische Erfahrungen. Z Kardiol 77, Suppl 1: 28

17. Hombach V, Höher M, Arnold G, Osypka P, Kochs M, Eggeling T, Höpp Hw, Hirche H, Hilger HH (1987) Die Hochfrequenzangioplastie – eine neue Methode zur Rekanalisation verschlossener arterieller Gefäße. CorVas 2: 67

18. Jungbluth A, Düber C, Rumpelt HJ, Erbel R, Meyer J (1988) Koronararterienmorphologie nach perkutaner transluminaler Koronarangioplastie (PTCA) mit Hämoperikard. Z Kardiol 77: 125

19. Kaltenbach M, Kober G, Scherer D (1980) Mechanische Dilatation von Koronararterienstenosen (Transluminale Angioplastie). Z Kardiol 69: 1

20. Keogh BE, Crea F, Pashazadeh M, Blackie RAS, Taylor KM (1988) Metal-capped optical fibres: is blood embolization a problem? In: Advances in Laser Medicine I, ecomed, Landsberg 236

21. Kober G, Hopf R, Reinemer H, Kaltenbach M (1985) Langzeitergebnisse der transluminalen koronaren Angioplastie von chronischen Herzkranzverschlüssen. Z Kardiol 74: 309

22. Leyser LJ, Bundy MA, Abreo F, Hanley HG, Fadely D, Walker JM (1986) Evaluation of coronary lysing system: results of a preclinical safety and efficacy study. Cath Cardiovasc Diag 12: 246

23. Matthews BJ, Ewels CJ, Kent KM (1988) Coronary dissection: a predictor of restenosis? Am Heart J 115: 547

24. McDonald RG, Panusch RS, Pepine CJ (1987) Rationale for use of glucocorticoids in modification of restenosis after percutaneous transluminal coronary angioplasty. Am J Cardiol 60: 56B

25. Kensey KR, Nash JE, Abrahams C, Zarins CK (1987) Recanalization of obstructed arteries with a flexible, rotating tip catheter. Radiology 165: 387

26. Meyer J, Schmitz H, Erbel R, Kiesslich T, Böcker-Josephs B, Krebs W, Braun PL, Bardos S, Minale C, Messmer BJ, Effert S (1981) Treatment of unstable angina pectoris with percutaneous transluminal coronary angioplasty. Cath Cardiovasc Diagn 7: 361

27. Meyer J, Erbel R, Pop T, Rupprecht HJ (1987) Derzeitiger Stand der intrakoronaren Ballondilatation. Internist 28: 736

28. Ritchie JL, Hansen DD, Intlekofer MJ, Hall M, Auth CD (1987) Rotational approaches to atherectomy and thrombectomy. Z Kardiol 76: 59

29. Rupprecht HJ, Erbel R, Brennecke R, Pop T, Jung D, Kottmeyer M, Hering R, Meyer J (1988) Aktuelle Komplikationsrate der perkutanen transluminalen Koronarangioplastie bei stabiler und unstabiler Angina. Dtsch med Wschr 113: 409

30. Schwartz L, Bourassa MG, Lespérance J, Aldridge HE, Kazin F, Salvatori VA, Henderson M, Bonan R, David PR (1988) Aspirin and dipyradimole in the prevention of restenosis after percutaneous transluminal coronary angioplasty. New Engl J Med 318: 1714

31. Serruys PW, Umans V, Heyndrickx GR, v.d. Brand M, De Feyter PJ, Wijns W, Jaski B, Hugenholtz PG (1985) Elective PTCA of totally occluded coronary arteries not associated with acute myocardial infarction; short-term and long-term results. Eur Heart J 6: 2

32. Shiu MF, Silverton NP, Oakley D, Cumberland D (1985) Acute coronary occlusion during percutaneous transluminal coronary angioplasty. Br Heart J 54: 129

33. Simpson JB, Selmon MR, Robertson GC, Cipriano PR, Hayden WG, Johnson DE, Fogarty TJ (1988) Transluminal atherectomy for occlusive peripheral vascular disease. Am J Cardiol 61: 96G

34. Slager CJ, Hugenholtz PG, Bom N, Lancée CT, Schuurbiers JCH, Serruys PW (1988) Spark erosion: an alternative to laser recanalisation. In: Advances in Laser Medicine I, ecomed, Landsberg 244

35. Steffenino G, Meier B, Finci L, Velebit V, von Segesser L, Faidutti B, Rutishauser W (1988) Acute

complications of elective coronary angioplasty: a review of 500 consecutive procedures. Br Heart J 59: 151
36. Vallbracht C, Schweitzer M, Kress J, Bamberg W, Kollath J, Liermann D, Paasch C, Rauber K, Roth FJ, Prignitz J, Beinborn W, Landgraf H, Breddin HK, Schoop W, Kaltenbach M (1988) Rotationsangioplastik – Erste klinische Ergebnisse bei peripheren Gafäßverschlüssen. Z Kardiol 77: 352
37. Vallbracht C, Krens J, Schweitzer W, Schneider M, Wendt Th, Ziemen M, Kollath J, Bamberg W, Kaltenbach M (1987) Rotationsangioplastik – ein neues Verfahren zur Gefäßeröffnung und -erweiterung. Experimentelle Befunde. Z Kardiol 76: 608
38. Whitworth HB, Roubin GS, Hollman J, Meier B, Leimgruber PP, Douglas JS, King SB, Gruentzig AR (1986) Effect of nifedipine on recurrent stenosis after percutaneous transluminal coronary angioplasty. J Am Coll Cardiol 8: 1271

Author's address:
Raimund Erbel, Prof. Dr. FACC FESC
II. Medical Clinic
Johannes Gutenberg-University
Langenbeckstr. 1
6500 Mainz, FRG

Recanalization of Chronic Total Occlusions: Results and Complications

C. W. Hamm and W. Bleifeld

Medical Clinic, Department of Cardiology, University Hospital Eppendorf, Hamburg, FRG

Introduction

Percutaneous transluminal coronary angioplasty (PTCA) was originally limited by Grüntzig to proximal isolated stenoses [3]. Based on growing experience of the operators and considerable improvement of the equipment the indication of PTCA has been extended to patients with double- or triple-vessel disease. Currently, several multi-center studies are being carried out to investigate the role of PTCA in multivessel disease [8]. One of the major preliminary results of the German multi-center trial (GABI) is that a major preclusion of PTCA in these patients is an occluded vessel requiring revascularization [6].

In contrast to high-grade stenoses or functional occlusions, the success rate with conventional angioplasty equipment in chronic total occlusions is in the range of only 40% to about 60% [1, 7, 10–15]. Recently, however, new angioplasty devices have been introduced which promise a higher success rate due to their special performance [5].

Recanalizations are considered to be low-risk procedures. First results are now available to answer the important question of whether complications remain at a low level with the new equipment.

The approach to total occlusions

The major determinant of the success of PTCA in total occlusions is the duration of the occlusion [10, 12]. Within the first month the success may reach 70% [12]. If the occluding thrombus becomes progressively organized the success falls to 50% within 6 months and to about 10% thereafter [12].

These results are obtained when a stiff guide wire is used and the balloon or a reper-

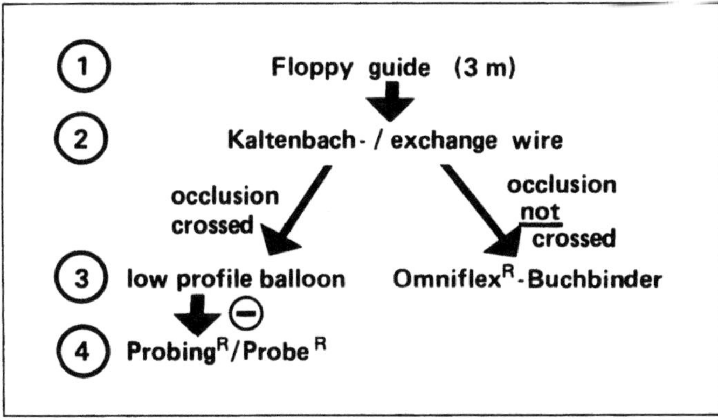

Fig. 1. Strategy to recanalize chronic total occlusions.

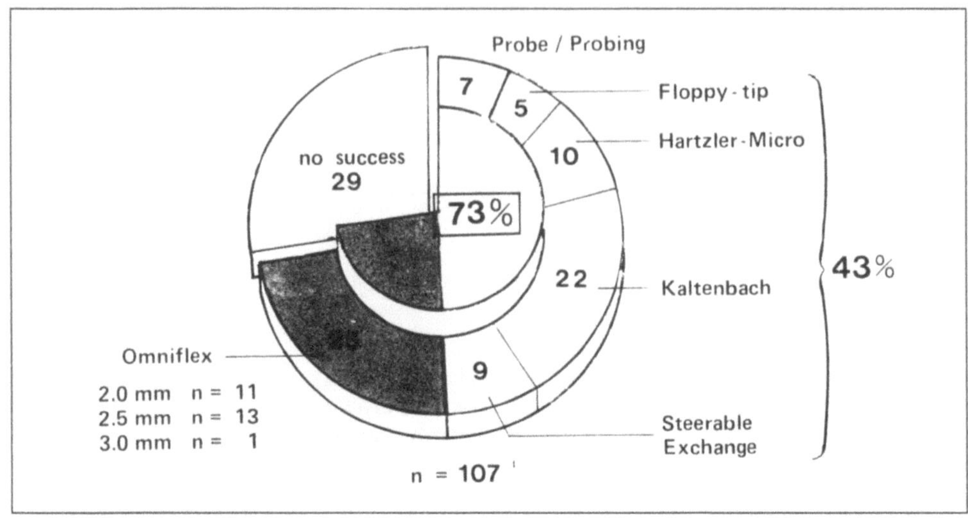

Fig. 2. Results obtained in 107 consecutive patients with conventional systems (43% success), and with the Probe/Probing system and the Buchbinder-Omniflex catheter.

fusion catheter [15] is advanced to the lesion for stabilization. In our institution this approach is successful in 46/107 (43%) consecutive chronic total occlusions (> 4 weeks–56 weeks duration).

If the conventional technique fails, our policy to continue depends on the success to cross the lesion by a guide wire (Fig. 1). When it was possible to penetrate the occlusion by a wire but not by a low-profile balloon, the wire is exchanged for a Probing (USCl/ Billerica, Massachusetts, USA) catheter, which is placed with the tip in the lesion. The Probing catheter serves as a sheath for the Probe (1-cm tip) balloon. In all seven (7%) such situations this approach was successful (Fig. 2).

For occlusions that cannot be crossed, even with stiffer wires, we take the Omniflex-Buchbinder (Medtronic, Minneapolis, USA) catheter. This catheter (first version) has a spring body for high pushability and good torque-control. The tip can be deflected from an external handle and so be directed into the correct lumen. In 25 of 54 cases the Omniflex system managed to open the occluded vessel, raising the total success rate to 73% (78/107 patients) (Fig. 2). This could regularly be achieved by gently pushing the catheter without any forceful maneuver. Sometimes, slow rotation of the entire system allows to "drill" the catheter into the lesion.

Complications in recanalization of total occlusions

Recanalizations of chronic total occlusions are generally considered to be low-risk procedures. The most critical complication of PTCA – the complete vessel occlusion – cannot occur. However, the occlusion of major side branches warrants attention and may require surgical back up. We observed this in one patient (1%) (Fig. 3a–c), who was sent to immediate bypass-surgery.

The most serious complication during the recanalization attempt is the perforation of the coronary artery wall. In our and other large series a penetration of an artery wall was not observed. Apparently, the coronary vessel wall is rather strong and this complication

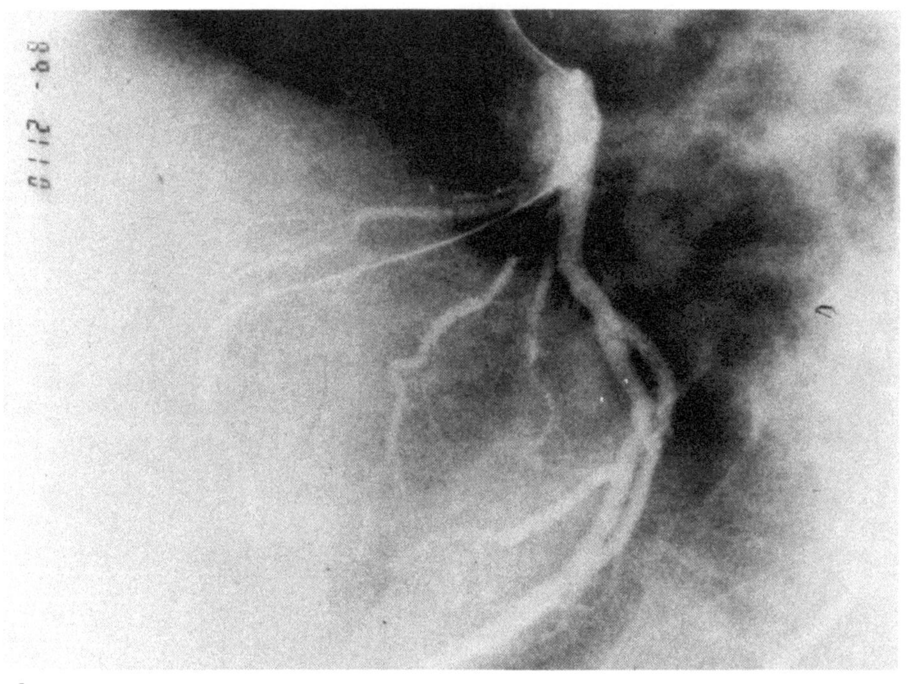

a

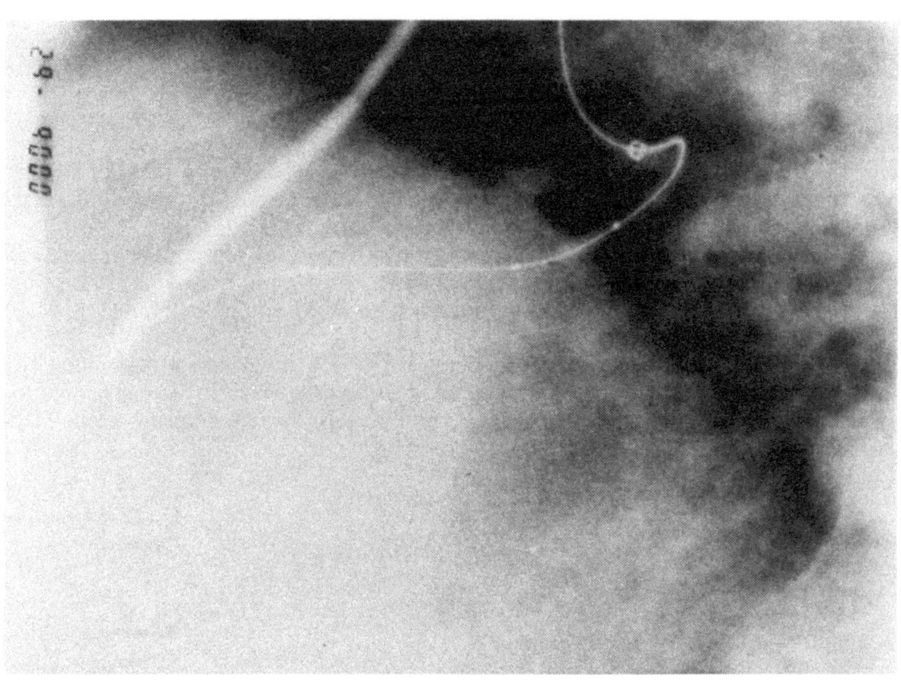

b

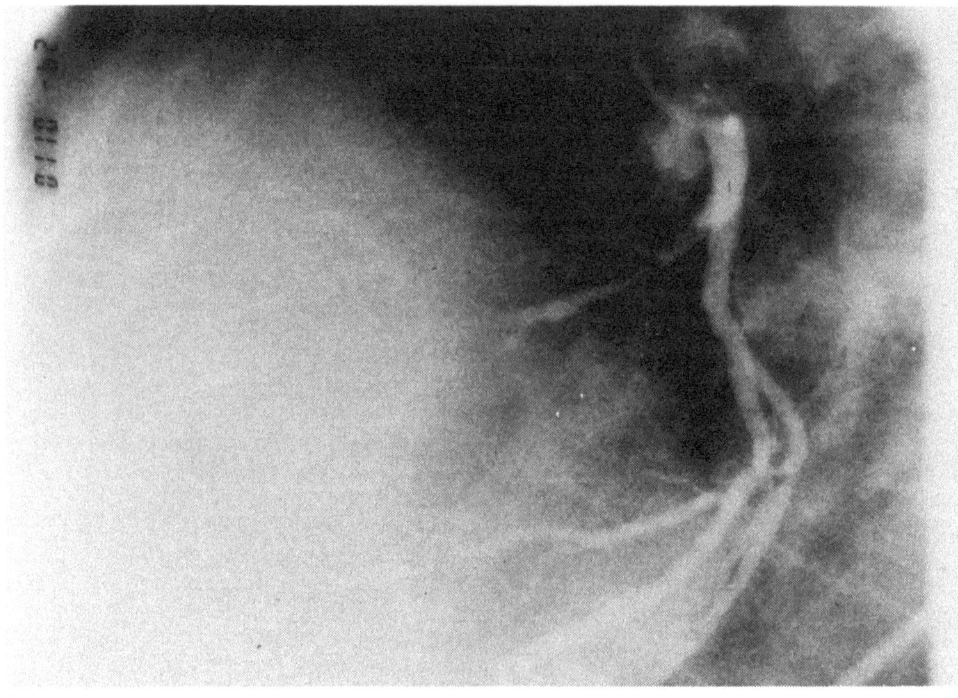

c

Fig. 3a–c. a) Total occlusion of the left anterior descending artery crossed by a guide wire; b) balloon inflation in lesion; c) occlusion of the first diagonal branch and fresh thrombotic material in the recanalized LAD. The patient developed acute angina and was sent to immediate bypass-surgery.

will only be seen after extremely vigorous maneuveurs. However, to better control bleeding after potential perforation we give only 5000 E heparin at the beginning of the procedure and another 10 000 E after the lesion is crossed.

More frequent are minor, subintimal dissections which require to terminate or postpone the procedure. Longer (> 2 cm) dissections have been observed in two cases (2%) of our series, one with the conventional approach and one with the Omniflex-balloon (Fig. 4a–c). Both patients had an uneventful follow-up.

However, complications like distal embolization [10, 13] and guide wire fracture [13] have been reported. The only other complication we observed was ventricular fibrillation after crossing the occlusion with a wire, probably induced through entering a small side branch (Table 1).

Table 1. Complications in recanalization of chronic total occlusions

● perforation	extremely rare
● long dissections	2%
● occlusion of side branches	1%
● distal embolization	190
● guide wire fracture	< 0.5%
● puncture site complications	1–2%
● emergency bypass surgery	< 1.0%

72

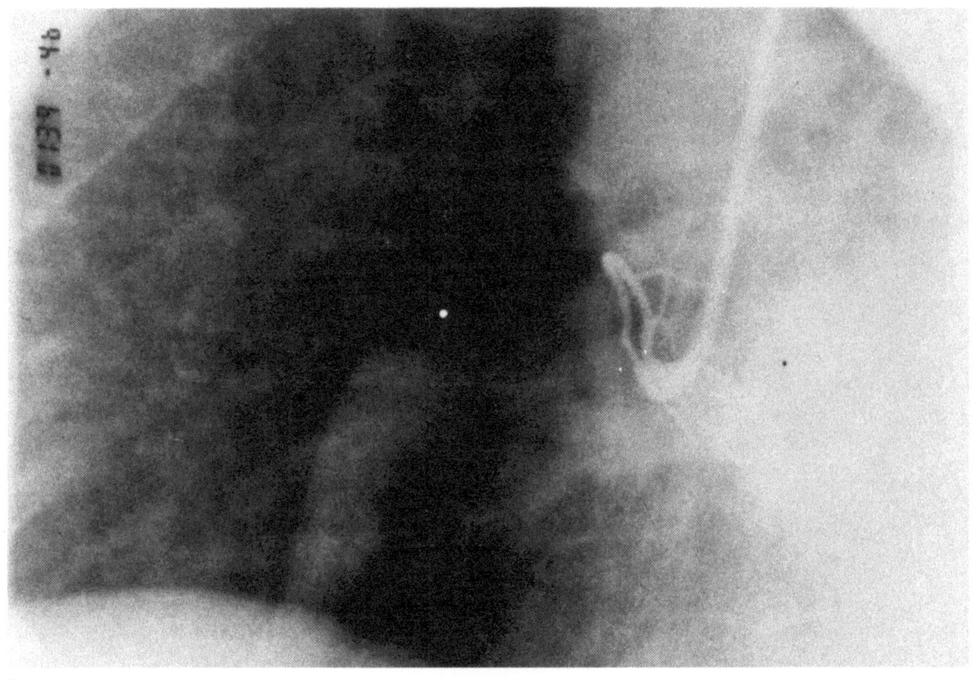

a

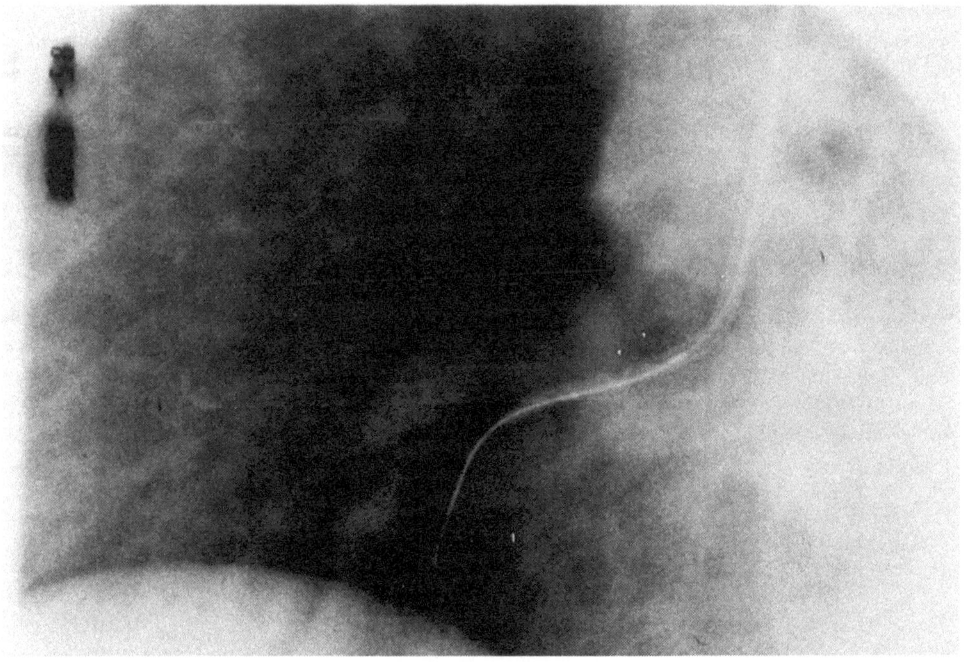

b

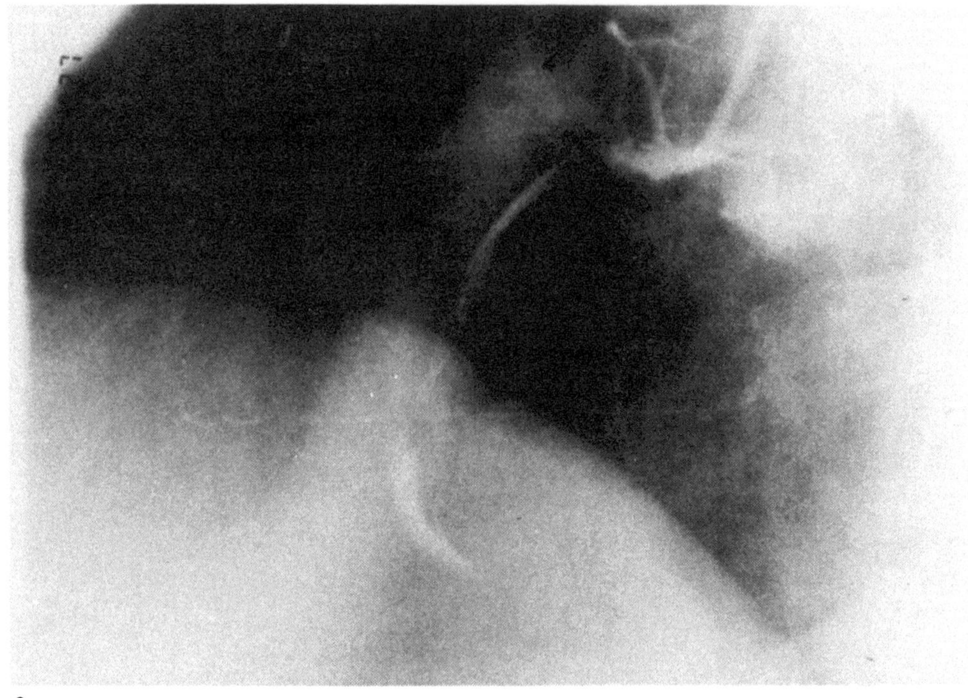

c

Fig. 4a–c. a) Proximal occlusion of the right coronary artery; b) inflation of a 2.0 mm Omniflex balloon; c) large subintimal dissection; the patient remained asymptomatic.

Even though it is a low risk procedure, recanalization should not be left to an inexperienced investigator. To avoid perforation or other complications a clearly defined protocol should be established in each laboratory.

Conclusion

With advanced angioplasty equipment successful recanalization can be achieved in 73% of chronic total occlusions. Recanalizations remain low-risk procedures when handled with experienced care, requiring acute surgical interventions in less than 1%. Further techniques like laser, radiofrequency or mechanical drills, which are currently under investigation, remain to be evaluated.

References

1. Dervan JP, Baim DS, Cherniles J, Grossman W (1983) Transluminal angioplasty of occluded coronary arteries: use of a movable guide wire system. Circulation 68, 4: 776–784
2. Ellis SG, Shaw RE, Gershony G, Thomas R, Roubin GS, Douglas JS, Topol EJ, Stertzer SH, Myler RK, King III SB (1989) Risk factors, time course and treatment effect for restenosis after successful percutaneous transluminal coronary angioplasty of chronic total occlusion. Am J Cardiol 63: 897–901
3. Grüntzig A (1978) Transluminal dilatation of coronary–artery stenosis Letter; Lancet 4: 263

4. Guidelines for percutaneous transluminal coronary angioplasty. (1988) Circulation 78: 486–502
5. Hamm CW, Schofer J, Kupper W (1988) Improved recanalization of coronary occlusions with a new catheter system. Circulation (Suppl II) 78, 4: 83
6. Hamm CW, Schuchert A, Bleifeld W, Ischinger TH, Delius W, Erbel R, Rupprecht HJ, Meyer J, Uebis R, Rudolph W (1989) Welcher Anteil der Patienten mit Mehr-Gefäß-Erkrankung eignet sich zur PTCA? Z Kardiol 78, Suppl 1
7. Holmes DR, Vlietstra RE (1985) Angioplasty in total coronary arterial occlusion. Herz 10: 292–297
8. Ischinger T, Hamm CW, Schuchert A, Bleifeld W (1989) Randomized comparison of PTCA versus coronary bypass surgery in patients with multivessel disease: The German Angioplasty Bypass Surgery Investigation (GABI) Europ Heart J, in press
9. Kaltenbach M (1984) Neue Technik zur steuerbaren Ballondilatation von Kranzgefäßverengungen Z Kardiol 73: 669–673
10. Kereiakes DJ, Selmon MR, McAuley BJ, McAuley DB, Sheehan DJ, Simpson JB (1985) Angioplasty in total coronary artery occlusion: Experience in 76 consecutive Patients. J Am Coll Cardiol 6: 526–33
11. Kober G, Hopf R, Reinemer H, Kaltenbach M (1985) Langzeitergebnisse der transluminalen koronaren Angioplastie von chronischen Herzkranzgefäßverschlüssen. Z Kardiol 74: 309–316
12. Melchior JP, Meier B, Urban P, Finci L, Steffenino G, Noble J, Rutishauser W (1987) Percutaneous transluminal coronary angioplasty for chronic total coronary arterial occlusion. Am J Cardiol 59: 535–538
13. Safian RD, McCabe CH, Sipperly ME, McKay RG, Baim DS (1988) Initial success and long-term follow-up of percutaneous transluminal coronary angioplasty in chronic total occlusions versus conventional stenoses. Am J Cardiol 61: 23G–28G
14. Serruys PW, Umans V, Heyndrickx GR, Brand M, Feyter PJ, Wuns W, Jaski B, Hugenholtz PG (1985) Elective PTCA of totally occluded coronary arteries not associated with acute myocardial infarction; short-term and long-term results. Europ Heart J 6: 2–12
15. Sievert H, Köhler KP, Kober G, Kaltenbach M (1988) Eröffnung chronischer Koronararterienverschlüsse mit einem Rekanalisationskatheter. Dtsch Med Wschr 113: 1703–1707

Author's address:
PD Dr. C.W. Hamm
II. Medizinische Klinik
Abteilung für Kardiologie
Universitätskrankenhaus Eppendorf
Martinistraße 52
2000 Hamburg 20, FRG

Complications in Conventional and New Angioplasty Techniques

M. Höher, V. Hombach, M. Kochs, W. Haerer, A. Schmidt, T. Eggeling

Department of Cardiology-Pneumonology-Angiology, University of Ulm, FRG

Introduction

The purpose of this article is to review the success rates and complication rates of balloon angioplasty, the conventional angioplasty technique, and newer techniques such as laser, atherectomy, and radiofrequency angioplasty. The main problem of such an analysis is the inhomogeneity of the so-called new interventional techniques in terms of both technical principles (thermal angioplasty by laser or radiofrequency, photoablation, mechanical atherectomy) and stage of development (Table 1). With some of the new techniques such as the Simpson atherectomy device [68, 76] clinical studies of about 500 patients are available, allowing a preliminary comparison with balloon angioplasty; other techniques such as radiofrequency angioplasty [34] have been clinically performed only in small patient groups.

As in other therapeutic procedures, success rates and complication rates of balloon angioplasty showed a typical time-course since its first use in 1977 by Grüntzig [25], which is characterized by both the development of operational skills and improvement of technology. Therefore, when comparing the success and complication rates of the newer angioplasty techniques with those of balloon dilatation (Table 2), it has to be borne in mind that most of the new techniques are in the developmental stage, i.e., where Grüntzig was in 1977. However, the ongoing comparison of the success rates of the newer technique to today's results of balloon dilatation are necessary, because the existing knowledge about the interdependence of success and complication rates of angioplasty proceures to certain clinical factors (single- vs multiple-vessel lesion, stable vs unstable angina, acute myocardial infarction) can be used to improve the selection process and the new technology itself, thus allowing a reasonable performance of all new angioplasty techniques.

Balloon dilatation

From the beginning in 1977, the number of balloon angioplasty procedures markedly increased from about 3000 between 1977 and 1982 to nearly 200 000 per year in the USA, and to about 13 000 per year in the FRG. During its first few years, PTCA was applied primarily to single, discrete lesions (75%), but now it is performed in several subsets of patients with double- (32%) or triple-vessel (22%) disease [11]. As shown by data of the U.S. National Heart, Lung, and Blood Institute Registry, in which 1155 patients undergoing PTCA between 1977 and 1981 were compared to 1802 patients treated by balloon angioplasty in 1985–1986, acute success rates defined as stenosis reduction of more than 20% increased from 69% to 89% in single-vessel disease and from 61%/66% to 86%/88% in double/triple-vessel disease [12]. Overall success rates measured as a reduction of at least 20% in all lesions attempted without death, myocardial infarction, or coronary bypass surgery significantly increased from 61% to 78% (Fig. 1). In a follow-up study of the same registry it was shown that the improved initial results reported in the 1985–1986 group were maintained at 1-year follow-up [13]. Interestingly, an angina-free status at 1 year was reported by 72% of the surviving patients, regardless of the initial success.

Table 1. New angioplasty techniques.

Laser	– Thermoablation (argon, Nd:YAG) – Indirect thermal effects (hot tip, heated balloon) – Photoablation (UV, excimer)
Radiofrequency	– Thermoablation – Indirect thermal effects (hot tip, heated balloon)
Atherectomy	– Cutting and extracting (Simpson) – High speed rotation (Auth) – Low speed rotation

During the last 2 years several studies have been published concerning factors affecting acute and long-term success of PTCA, which shall be shortly discussed in the following in terms of complications (Table 3).

Operational skills

It is well accepted that operational skills of the individual physicians performing PTCA are important for the result of the procedure, but there is only little data available about this issue, although the above-mentioned improvement of success rates mostly reflects the learning curve of all operators. Jacob et al. [37] showed in a group of 6 physicians, who had performed 131 PTCA in 1983/84, and 279 in 1984/85, a significant increase of the success rate from 76% to 84%, accompanied by a decrease of coronary occlusions from 8.4% to 5.7%, and a decrease of emergency bypass surgery from 11% to 5.4%.

From the same laboratory the 1986–1987 experience was recently reported [28]. Comparing physicians with a case load of more than 100 procedures per year to those with less than 100 per year, they found that success rates with simple lesions were similar for both

Table 2. Overall complication rates of balloon angioplasty from the NHLBI registry for 1985–1986.

Complications of Coronary Angioplasty (n = 1.801)	%
Coronary spasm	1.3
Coronary occlusion	4.9
Coronary dissection	4.8
Prolonged angina	4.7
Death	1.0
Nonfatal infarction	4.3
Emergency CABG	3.5
Death, MI or emergency CABG	7.2

(from: Holmes DR et al, JACC 12: 1149–1155, 1988)

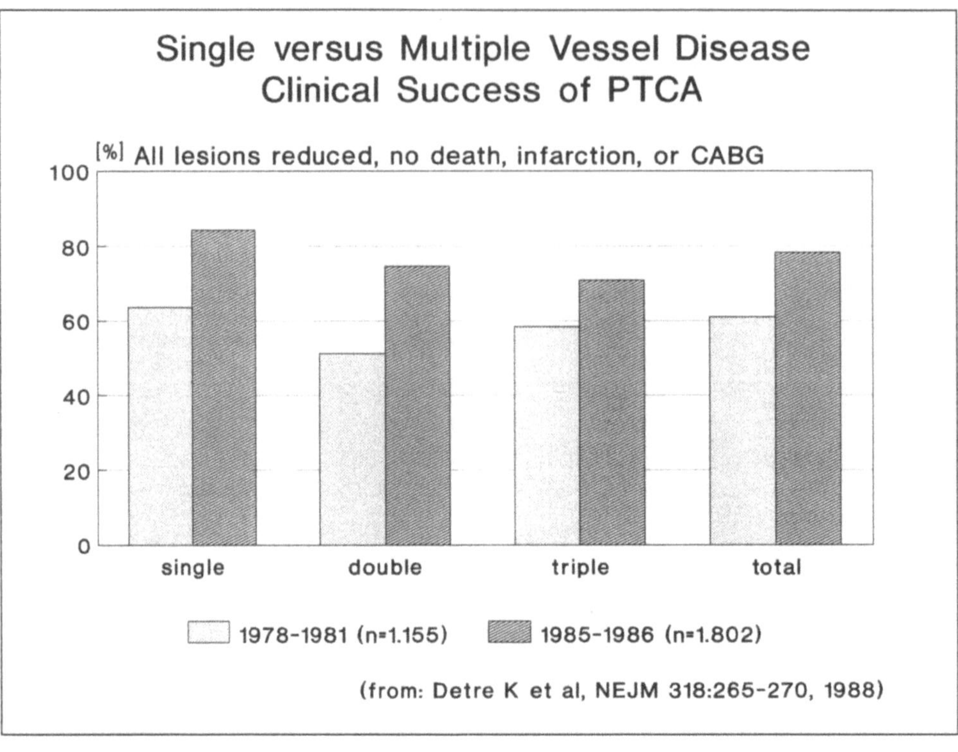

Fig. 1. Clinical success rates in single, double, and triple vessel disease according to the U.S. National Heart, Lung, and blood Institute Registry. Clinical success was defined as reduction by at least 20% of all attempted stenosis without death, myocardial infarction or emergency bypass surgery.

groups (93% vs 90%), but in complicated lesions involving a bifurcation or those with marked eccentricity, calcifiction or ulceration the success rate of the high frequency operators was significantly better (81%) as compared to the low frequency operators (69%). In parallel the more experienced physicians had a clearly lower complication rate (3.1% vs 7.5%), although the percentage of complex lesions was greater (41% vs 33%). Comparing the three periods 1983–1987 in both physician groups, Hamad et al. [28] found that the high-frequency operators improved their overall success rate from 86% to 91%, despite changes in patient selection, whereas in the low-frequency operator group success rate remained nearly constant (83% to 84%). Complication rates were reduced by both groups during these 4 years to half of the initial percentage (5.6% to 2.8% vs 9.0% to 4.4%), which may be due to both individual learning curves and technical developments. Nevertheless, this data shows that about 50% of complication rates may be assumed to be operator-related, a fact which is often not mentioned.

Technical factors

A major factor for reduction of complications and increase of success rates was the introduction of independently movable guidewires in 1982 that could be reshaped and

Table 3. Complications of PTCA – specific factors.

- **■** Time course
  - operator's skill
  - improvement of technology

- **■** Single versus multiple vessel disease

- **■** Single lesion versus multiple lesion dilatation

- **■** Stage of coronary heart disease
  - stable/unstable angina
  - acute myocardial infarction

- **■** Individual risk factors
  - age
  - gender
  - collateral status

directed to the vessel approached [69]. Using this system the primary success rates of the first 50–70 procedures of an individual operator, which were 50–64% [25, 3], using fixed guidewire systems, increased to more than 90% [30]. Other factors were improvements in guiding catheters and low-profile balloons, as well as the use of low-osmolality contrast media [31]. Balloon size has been shown to have a great influence on complication rate. Since there were some data indicating that a low balloon-to-artery diameter ratio is predictive of restenosis, Roubin et al. [59] started a prospective randomized study in 336 patients, comparing larger and smaller balloons. In this study, which was halted at the time when clinically important differences in acute complications emerged, emergency bypass graft surgery (usually for treatment of vessel dissection) was required in 7.1% of patients with a larger balloon (balloon-to-artery diameter ratio 1.13), but only in 3.6% of patients with a smaller balloon size (balloon-to-artery diameter ratio 0.93). Additionally, myocardial infarction complicated 7.7% of procedures in which large balloons were assigned, but only 3.0% of procedures in the smaller balloon group. Initial stenosis reduction and restenosis rate (44% vs 39%) did not differ between both groups, indicating that oversizing of balloons will result in increased complications, particularly in patients with multivessel disease or complex lesion morphology.

Multiple- vs single-vessel disease

Multivessel disease may also be appropriately treated by balloon dilatation. Although there are large studies reporting a 90% success rate and a 95% clinical improvement in multivessel disease, which is quite similar to the results in single-vessel disease [53, 36, 43], there is evidence from other studies that the overall in-hospital mortality is dependent on the extent of vessel disease, and that the frequency of nonfatal complications increases with an increased number of vessels attempted [33, 12, 16].

Analysing the results of PTCA in multiple-vessel disease, the effect of single lesion PTCA in single- vs double- or triple-vessel disease should be mentioned separately from the results of multilesion PTCA procedures with one vs two or more lesions attempted. From the data of the NHLBI Angioplasty Registry the percentage of PTCA in patients with double or triple vessel disease increased from 25% in 1977–1981 to 53% in 1985–1986 [12]. It is remarkable that in between both time periods studied the angiographic success rates by lesions did not differ very much in single- as compared to double- or triple-vessel disease (1977–1981: single 69%, double/triple 61%/66%; 1985–1986: single 89%, double/triple 86%/88%). Success was defined in the NHLBI report as 20% stenosis reduction. This definition is less rigid than the more commonly used of a residual stenosis less than 50% in diameter.

In contrast to the quite similar results in single-, double- or triple-vessel disease, the number of lesions treated has a significant influence on the success rate. In the NHLBI registry the number of multiple lesion PTCA increased from 8% in 1977–1981 to 50% in 1985–1986. Clinical success, defined as reduction by more than 20% of all lesions for which procedures were attempted, and no death, infarction or bypass surgery, was 84% in single-, but 71% in triple-vessel procedures (Fig. 1). Gaul et al. [22] recently showed that in multilesion PTCA there is no difference in success rates between multivessel multilesion and single-vessel multilesion PTCA. Therefore, in terms of succes rates, the number of lesions attempted in a single patient seems to be much more important than the number of diseased vessels in a patient. In terms of complications both multivessel disease and multilesion procedures seem to be independent risk factors.

From the NHLBI data there is evidence that in-hospital mortality increases with the number of diseased vessels (Table 3). In the NHLBI registry mortality was 0.2% in single-, 0.9% in double- and 2.2% in triple-vessel disease [33]. There were nonsignificant trends toward higher rates of nonfatal myocardial infarction and emergency coronary artery bypass grafting in patients with more severe disease. The incidence of the combined outcome of death, myocardial infarction or emergency bypass surgery increased from 5.5% in single to 9.3% in triple-vessel disease (Table 4).

Evidence for an increased complication rate with more severe vessel disease was also found for vessel occlusion and prolonged angina. Other complications such as spasm, dissection, branch occlusion, ventricular fibrillation, and abrupt closure occurred at rates that were independent of the extent of vessel disease. According to the number of vessels in which dilatation was attempted, it was found that the frequency of nonfatal infarction increases with an increased number of vessels attempted (4.1% vs 7.3% for attempts at one and three vessels). In contrast, Gaul et al. [22] reported that in 714 patients with multilesion PTCA the incidence of acute occlusion was relatively low and quite similar in multilesion single vessel (3.3%) and multilesion multivessel procedures (2.9%).

These percentages are similar to the incidence of acute occlusion in series of patients undergoing predominantly single-vessel angioplasty reported by other authors (2.1% to 4.4%) [32, 16, 67]. But since in multivessel angioplasty more than one vessel may simultaneously occlude, acute occlusion in such cases has a higher complication rate. In the study of Gaul et al. [22] the maximal increase in creatine kinase after acute occlusion

Table 4. Comparison of complications of balloon angioplasty in single-, double- and triple-vessel disease, from the NHLBI registry. In double- and triple-vessel disease complications are significantly more frequent.

	Vessel disease		
	Single	Double	Triple
Death	0.2	0.9	2.2%
Nonfatal MI	3.5	5.2	5.2%
Emergency CABG	2.9	3.9	4.4%
Death, MI or emergency CABG	5.5	8.1	9.3%
Occlusion	3.9	4.5	7.9%
Prolonged angina	3.5	5.2	6.5%

(from: Holmes DR et al., JACC 12, 1988)

during multilesion PTCA was significantly higher in the multivessel (1.700 U/l) as compared to the single-vessel group (563 U/l). Emergency bypass surgery was necessary in 50% of patients with acute occlusion following multivessel angioplasty, but only in 8% following multilesion, single-vessel angioplasty. A large intimal tear and hypotension seem to be important predisposing factors to the acute occlusion syndrome [22, 16, 32, 33].

In multilesion dilation, hypotension bears an additional risk since frequently the first artery closes when hypotension is induced during the second vessel attempt [22]. For this reason, if the first angioplasty results in a large intimal tear or the patient is relatively hypotensive, the procedure might be safer if the second vessel angioplasty is deferred to another day. Although the overall incidence of any specific complication of balloon dilatation is low, complications tend to occur in clusters. Holmes et al. reported that procedure-related ventricular fibrillation, although occurring in only 21/1801 patients (1.2%), was associated with a 14% mortality and a 48% incidence of nonfatal infarction.

Repeat balloon dilatation

The high incidence of restenosis after primary balloon dilatation of 12% to 37% is one of the major unsolved problems of this kind of treatment [50, 39]. During recent years the number of repeat angioplasties due to restenosis continuously increased to about 18% of the procedures [13]. Repeat angioplasty for restenosis following primarily successful balloon dilatation is more sucessful and less dangerous than the initial procedure. Meier et al. [52] reported a 97% primary success rate of repeat angioplasty, compared to 85% of the initial procedure. A similar difference was found by Williams et al. [77], who had a 61% primary success rate in the initial procedure and a 85% success rate during repeat angioplasty. This "improvement" of success rate in repeat angioplasty can be easily explained by case selection. Only those lesions qualify for repeat angioplasty that have been successfully dilated before, and patients whose initial angioplasty was complicated will less often be chosen for a repeat procedure. Follow-up studies after PTCA have shown that patients who developed intermittent acute closure during the initial procedure have a much higher morbidity and mortality within the first year. The NHLBI registry data show that even though patients comprise only 7% of the cohort, nearly 20% of the 1-year mortality, nearly 40% of all infarctions, and nearly 25% of all coronary bypass operations occurred in this small subset [13].

Since repeat angioplasty is much less frequent in this group with complications after the initial angioplasty, there is a positive selection process that results in a patient group of lower risk at repeat angioplasty as compared to the patient group undergoing the initial procedure.

The same good results described for second angioplasty seems to be achievable in following angioplasties. Teirstein et al. [74] reported a 93% procedural success rate in 74 patients, in whom a third angioplasty was performed due to second restenosis, and they reported a 94% procedural success rate in 16 patients with fourth angioplasty due to third restenosis. Severe procedural complications were reported by Teirstein et al. [74] in 7% during third angioplasty and in 6% (1/16) during fourth angioplasty. At third angioplasty 3/74 patients (4%) required emergency bypass surgery and 2 patients (3%) died, since they were deemed inoperable. Since, in the study of Teirstein, all severe complications occured in patients suffering from double- or triple-vessel disease, complication rates of repeat angioplasty were not different from those of primary angioplasty. (From the NHLBI registry, emergency surgery rate is 3.9% (4.4%) and mortality is 0.9% (2.2%) in double- (triple-) vessel disease.)

Meier et al. [52] reported an even lower complication rate of a repeat procedure as compared to primary angioplasty. In 95 patients undergoing repeat (second) angioplasty due to restenosis, emergency surgery rate (1% vs 5%) and Q-wave infarction rate (0% vs 1%) were not significantly different from those in primary angioplasty. However, only 8% of patients with repeat angioplasty had one or more clinically significant complications, compared to 15% of the total cohort of 514 patients. The data of the American Registry, including 3079 initial and 203 repeat angioplasties, also showed significantly less myocardial infarctions (2% vs 5%), emergency operations (2% vs 7%), and death (0% vs 1%) during repeat angioplasty as compared to the initial procedures [77].

Bypass graft angioplasty

Primary success rate of angioplasty of bypass grafts is equal or even better than that of native arteries [50]. Douglas et al. [15] reported on 121 consecutive cases with prior bypass surgery, in which primary success rates of angioplasty were 94% at the distal anastomosis, 80% at the proximal anastomosis, and 96% within the graft body, as compared to a 83% primary success rate at the native arteries. Other studies found no differences of the success rates between the various locations in the graft [58], but restenosis is more frequent in graft bodies and proximal anastomoses than in distal anastomoses [15].

In an overview of Meier [50], summarizing 643 patients from 10 studies, primary success rate was 85% in patients with prior bypass surgery. Complication rates for death (1%), infarction (3%), and emergency surgery (2%) were comparable to primary angioplasties in patients without prior bypass surgery. Also, in a study of Ellis et al. [16] who analyzed 13 procedural deaths after acute vessel closure out of 8207 consecutive angioplasties, prior bypass surgery had no predictive value.

Dorros et al. [14] recently reported on 65 patients, in whom balloon dilatation was performed with 2–4 previous coronary bypass operations. In this higher risk patient group with prior myocardial infarction in 65% and ejection fraction below 35% in 17%, overall success rates were 88% in native coronaries and 83% in vein grafts. Differences of success rates between proximal anastomosis (79%), graft shaft (100%), and distal anastomosis (81%) were not significant, but comparing these data with the above-mentioned results of Douglas et al. [15], the best primary angioplasty results seem to be achievable in venous bypass shaft.

In the study of Dorros et al. [14] the mortality rate was 3%, emergency bypass surgery was necessary in 1%, and transmural myocardial infarction occurred in 1%.

A special complication of bypass graft angioplasty is distal embolization of atherosclerotic plaques and thrombotic material, which occurs in about 6% [14], typically with angioplasty of graft body stenoses [4]. Though embolization of small and not occlusive particles is likely to occur during most balloon procedures, this seems to become more relevant in bypass graft dilatation due to the caliber difference between the bypass graft and the native artery. The same problem is found in reopening thrombotically occluded venous bypass grafts. Due to the mass of thrombotic material within an acutely occluded bypass graft, thrombotic embolization is likely to occur. Therefore, intragraft streptokinase or urokinase during balloon dilatation of venous bypass grafts has been recommended [14, 58].

Angioplasty in acute myocardial infarction

At present there is a controversial discussion about the value of coronary angioplasty for acute myocardial infarction. During 1982 to 1986 several studies were published indicating that coronary angioplasty in evolving myocardial infarction is a relatively safe and successful therapy. Summarizing the results of angioplasty in acute myocardial infarction from 637 patients of 15 smaller studies, Meier [50] described a 92% primary success rate, a 5% in-hospital mortality, 4% vessel occlusions by angioplasty, and 15% reocclusions (7% with myocardial infarction). This in-hospital mortality rate of 5% is much lower than the 11–20% mortality rate in historical control groups treated with traditional conservative therapy, but the studies did not include all high risk patients, for example, those older than 70 years or with cardiogenic shock. Recent randomized trials comparing thrombolytic therapy alone to a combination of thrombolytic therapy and coronary angioplasty have not shown any benefit from angioplasty performed early in acute myocardial infarction [75, 66, 73]. In the TIMI-II trial that included 3262 patients, within 42 days the angioplasty group had a 5.2% mortality and a 6.4% infarction rate as compared to a 4.7% mortality and a 5.8% reinfarction rate in the group with conservative treatment using only rt-PA. Of the 878 patients, in whom angioplasty was performed in acute myocardial infarction, PTCA was successful in 94% of patent vessels and in 92% of occluded arteries, which is comparable to the procedural success rates of balloon dilatation in stable angina. Within 24 h after PTCA 7.7% of these patients had a total occlusion of the infarcted artery, 5.4% had reinfarction, 2.5% had emergency bypass surgery, and 0.5% died [73].

An additional major complication of combined thrombolysis and angioplasty is the high (15–29%) incidence of serious hemorrhage [55]. Since about 13% of patients with acute myocardial infarction present contraindictions to thrombolytic therapy and the failure rate for currently available thrombolytic agents is 25–65%, the main problem of angioplasty in acute infarction seems to be the definition of subgroups most probably profiting from early angioplasty.

In a recent study of 500 consecutive patients treated with coronary angioplasty for acute myocardial infarction, Ellis et al. [17] found an improved in-hospital survival for patients with cardiogenic shock or anterior myocardial infarction. In patients with anterior infarction and successful balloon dilatation mortality was significantly lower (7.2%) than in those with failed PTCA (36%). Though this indicates a positive effect of successful PTCA in acute anterior infarction, it has to be mentioned that the 36% mortality rate after unsuccessful procedures is higher than that reported from conservative treated series, suggesting possible harm from failed angioplasty. In patients with acute inferior infarction successful PTCA of the infarct-related vessel had no significant influence on mortality [17]. Beside the smaller amount of myocardium at risk in inferior myocardial infarction, development of ventricular fibrillation due to sudden reopening of the vessel, which is more likely in the right than in the left coronary artery, might be an explanation. From the NHLBI registry there is evidence that ventricular fibrillation shows a very strong association with mortality [33].

In contrast to the above-mentioned PTCA in addition to thrombolysis, O'Keefe et al. [54] recently reported about 500 ptients with acute myocardial infarction treated by coronary angioplasty without antecedent thrombolytic therapy. In this unselected patient group overall in-hospital mortality rate was 7.2%, which is comparable to the results achieved in the large thrombolysis trials (4–7%) [66, 73, 75] considering the rigid selection criteria of these studies. Using the same criteria, i.e., excluding patients over age 75, with prior bypass surgery, cardiogenic shock or symptoms lasting longer than 4 h, O'Keefe et al. [54] found an in-hospital mortality of only 1.8%. But, similar to the study of Ellis et al. [17], mortality was very high in patients with failed angioplasty (34.3%). Angioplasty success rates were 94% in native arteries and 83% in venous bypass grafts. Bleeding complications occurred in 3%, which is much lower than in angioplasty studies with additional thrombolytic therapy (15–29%). Reocclusion of the infarct-related artery was noted in 15% of 307 patients with angiographic follow-up before hospital discharge.

Cardiac death after elective coronary angioplasty in carefully selected patient groups is fortunately rare in experienced centers, occurring in 0.16–1.0% of patients [16]. From several studies there is evidence that, beside the above discussed presence of multivessel disease, collateral vessels emanating from the dilated vessel, age over 65 years, and female gender are independent preprocedural risk factors [16, 33]. Collateral vessels emanating from the dilated vessel enlarge the mass of myocardium at risk in case of acute closure of the vessel. Analyzing 13 cardiac deaths from 294 vessel closures following balloon dilatation, Ellis et al. [16] reported two deaths among four patients with collateral vessels who had dilation of the collateralized artery before dilation of the artery closed. Of the four patients who had the collateralizing vessel dilated first and developed acute closure, all four died.

At present the reasons for the higher complication rate in females are not fully understood. Female patients respond more frequently to vasodilators with hypotension, have a poorer contractile reserve, and volume depletion is more likely to occur in women, because they have a smaller intravascular volume. Hypotension, both after initial arteriography plus nitroglycerin and after acute vessel closure, has been identified as an independent risk factor [16]. In addition, women have smaller coronary vessels than do men [38]. Therefore, it has been suggested that the early standard use of 3.0 mm balloons, which were sometimes oversized for women, predisposed to acute closure.

Complications of new angioplasty techniques

During recent years various new angioplasty techniques have been developed on the basis of very different technical principles, such as laser, mechanical cutting, or thermal energy. Most of these new angioplasty techniques are in a developmental stage and have been used mainly in the peripheral arteries. With the exception of the Simpson atherectomy device, complication rates of the first coronary applications of these newer techniques are very preliminary and do not allow a comparison with the results and complications of balloon angioplasty.

Laser angioplasty. Thermoablation by continuous wave lasers

Laser angioplasty of coronary atherosclerotic tissue was initially described by Lee et al. [45]. In the early studies continuous wave lasers, such as the argon and the Nd : YAG laser coupled to a bare fiberoptic were used. Atherosclerotic tissue can be removed with such continuous wave lasers by photothermal ablation, histologically characterized by a cone-shaped crater surrounded by concentric zones of carbonized material, eosinophilic coagulum, and vacuolozation [26]. In 1984, Choy et al. [9] attempted the first bare fiber continuous-wave argon laser angioplasty of native coronary arteries at the time of bypass surgery. Under direct vision, 4/5 vessels were recanalized, but all vessels had reoccluded by 1 to 3 months. Mechanical perforation of the vessel wall occurred in one patient. In the following years several investigators studied the effects of direct continuous wave laser angioplasty in peripheral arteries without convincing results [23, 1]. The main limitations of these techniques were:
1) vascular perforations, because of mechanical trauma from the sharp exposed fiber tip and the nonaxial delivery of laser energy;
2) a high rate of vascular reocclusion as a result of the small diameter of the recanalized lumen (300–400 μm);

3) vascular spasm and pain occurring because of the thermally induced vasomotor reactivity.

After improvement of fiber technology, direct thermal laser angioplasty recently was used again in coronary arteries by three investigators. Côté et al. [10] used a pulsed argon laser and a fiberoptic catheter guided by a wire in five patients with high-grade coronary stenoses. Though he could slightly improve all targeted stenoses, significant residual stenoses (> 50%) remained in all cases. There were no complications, probably due to the guidewire technique. Foschi et al. [19] treated nine subtotal occlusions in eight patients (five native coronary arteries and four saphenous vein grafts) that could not be passed with a guidewire, using direct,continuous, argon laser application with an optical fiber and lens assembly that diverged the laser beam to 40°. There were no complications and laser treatment allowed subsequent penetration of the lesions with a guidewire, followed by balloon angioplasty.

Using the same argon laser system as Foschi et al. [19], Schömig et al. [65] could not reopen any of five occluded native coronary arteries, but observed marked pain in two of the five patients during laser application with subsequent ventricular fibrillation and development of a localized pericarditis in one patient.

Summarizing these studies, direct application of continuous wave laser energy in the coronaries may be useful to pass subtotal occlussions for subsequent balloon dilatation, but complication rate still seems to be high.

Excimer laser angioplasty

From experimental studies it is known that ultraviolet pulsed light from excimer lasers is superior to continuous wave argon or Nd: YAG lasers in terms of ablation of atherosclerotic tissue [26]. The three main advantages of excimer laser are:
1) tissue ablation without thermal injury to boundary tissue sites;
2) removal of calcified plaques;
3) energy delivery is restricted to a very close range, which reduces the risk of perforation.

Although exact mechanisms of ablation by excimer lasers remain to be elucidated, the high-energy ultraviolet photons remove tissue by the process of ablative photodecomposition [21]. Due to the marked attenuation of ultraviolet energy by fiber optics and the high peak power of the nanosecond laser pulses, transmission of the excimer light through fibers has been the main problem of this technique [47].

During the last years several initial clinical studies including a total of more than 100 patients have shown the feasibility of excimer laser angioplasty of coronary lesions [6, 40, 48, 49] (Table 5). In the initial report, Litvack et al. [48] successfully treated four lesions in two patients without complications, reaching a mean stenosis reduction from 77% to 22.5%, without additional balloon dilation and complications. Margolis et al. [49] (from the same group) reported a successful stenosis reduction (> 20%) in 76% of 41 patients, in whom 53 lesions were treated. Achieving a mean stenosis reduction by laser alone from 89% to 50%, they performed additional balloon dilatation in 85% of patients. Complications occurred in 7% of patients including one emergency bypass surgery, one occlussion with subsequent non-Q-infarction, and one dissection, but no vessel perforation. Karsch et al. [40] achieved a ≥ 20% stenosis reduction in 85% of 40 patients treated by excimer laser angioplasty, resulting in a mean stenosis reduction from 85% to 63%. Within their first five patients, three patients developed an intimal dissection at the distal end of the stenosis treated by laser during subsequent balloon dilatation. In contrast to the results of Litvack and Margolis, Karsch et al. [40] observed a 25% incidence of coronary spasms during excimer lasing. This might have been due to the somewhat lower power density of

Table 5. Coronary excimer laser angioplasty.

Author	Method	Pat. No.	Lesion No	Success Rate *	Compli- cation	Death	AMI	CABG	Other
Litvack 1989	XeCl Excimer	2	4	100% PTCA in 0/4	0%	0	0	0	–
Margolis 1989	XeCl Excimer	41	53	76% PTCA in 35/41	7%	0	1	1	1 dissection
Karsch 1989	XeCl Excimer	40	40	85% PTCA in 16/40	25%	0	0	0	3 dissections 25% spasms
Buchwald 1989	XeCl Excimer	17	17	100% PTCA in 10/17	6%	0	0	0	1 occlusion
Kochs 1990	XeCl Excimer	16	16	69% PTCA in 14/16	88%	0	0	0	5 dissections 4 occlusions 3 spasms 5 thrombi

* stenosis reduction ›20%

the excimer-fiber system used by Karsch et al. [40] as compared to that of the Los Angeles group, resulting in increased thermal effects.

Using the same excimer laser as Karsch et al. [40], Buchwald et al. [6] reported a $\geq 20\%$ stenosis reduction in all 17 patients treated with excimer angioplasty without any acute complications. In eight patients with complete coronary occlusions, residual stenosis after laser alone was $59 \pm 13\%$; in nine patients with high-grade coronary stenoses excimer laser angioplasty alone reached a stenosis reduction of $91 \pm 5\%$ to $49 \pm 7\%$. Subsequent PTCA was performed in 10/17 (59%) patients, in whom residual stenosis after excimer angioplasty was exceeded 50%.

Our group treated sixteen patients by excimer laser angioplasty, achieving a mean stenosis reduction from $75 \pm 10\%$ to $51 \pm 10\%$ with the same Technolas Max-10 laser as used by Karsch et al. [40] and Buchwald et al [6]. Additional balloon dilatation was performed in 14/16 patients. Complications of laser angioplasty were frequent, including five intimal dissections, four temporal vessel occlusions, three vascular spasms, and intracoronary thrombus formation in five patients. All these complications could be managed by conventional balloon dilatation (Kochs et al., in press).

Summarizing the initial clinical results of coronary excimer laser angioplasty, the introduction of excimer laser technology has solved several major problems (such as perforation of vessel) that were reported for previous continuous wave laser technology. At present, the complication rate of excimer angioplasty exceeds that of PTCA, although the former is mainly performed in selected patient groups. The clinical value of laser angioplasty still remains to be defined, since presently in most procedures, excimer angioplasty is followed by balloon dilatation. Further technical improvements, including larger or self-expandable laser catheters, are necessary to use excimer angioplasty as a stand-alone procedure and to allow a thorough comparison between balloon and laser angioplasty.

Table 6. Coronary thermal angioplasty.

Author	Method	Pat. No.	Lesion No	Success Rate	Compli- cation	Death	AMI	CABG	Other
Linne- meier 1989	argon laser- probe	19	22 *	95%	14%	0	1	0	1 embolism 1 sidebranch occlusion
Sanborn 1989	argon laser- probe	11	11 *	64%	27%	0	3	0	–
Hombach 1989	radio- fre- quency	13	13 *	77%	8%	0	0	0	1 occlusion
Spears 1989	laser- balloon	65	76 **	95% (after PTCA)	8%	0	0	0	1 dissection 1 embolism 1 aneurysm 2 vent. fibrill.

* stenosis reduction › 20%

** additional 30% increase of vessel diameter after PTCA

Thermal angioplasty. Hot-tip laser angioplasty

To overcome the problems with direct application of continuous wave laser energy onto the tissue, i.e., narrow laser beam resulting in a small lumen and a high perforation risk, laser catheters have been equipped with metal caps. In these "hot-tip" laser systems, laser is used as the energy source the heat the metal olive-like cap at the tip of the fiberoptic catheter. Experimental studies have demonstrated an improved safety and efficacy of these laser-heated probes, compared with bare fiberoptics, and less restenosis than with conventional balloon angioplasty [61, 62]. After successful application in peripheral arteries, coronary hot-tip laser angioplasty has now been performed in a limited number of patients. The main complications of intracoronary heat application were spasms and thrombus formation, which occurred more frequently in the coronary than in the larger femoral arteries (Table 6). Sanborn and Cumberland [63] reported on seven patients, in whom coronary laser hot-tip angioplasty was successful in four patients without any complications. In three patients the lesion could not be recanalized due to vessel tortuosity. In another group of four patients, three of four lesions could be crossed, but there were three myocardial infarctions [63]. Recently, Linnemeier et al. [46] reported a 95% procedural success rate of the laser probe in 22 coronary lesions of 19 patients. Complications related to spasm or thrombosis occurred in three vessels (14%), including one distal embolization, closure of a side branch vessel, and late closure of an LAD graft after 6 days. From in vitro studies there is evidence that relatively large debris particles up to 200–300 μm (4–5 per lasing) are formed during use of the hot-tip laser, which cause a potential embolization hazard [41, 56]. The amount of debris is energy- and blood-flow-dependent [42]. From our experience with the radiofrequency catheter, thrombus formation and vascular spasms are mainly caused by the relatively large lateral surface area of the metal tip of the hot-tip probes, resulting in heating of the blood and the vascular wall instead of the targeted atherosclerotic lesion. This view is supported by a recent report by Chan et al. [8], who used a new laserprobe (in which the laser energy is confined and localized to a tiny thermal band on the prominent shoulder of the probe) in two patients with totally occluded right coronary arteries. In both patients thermal laser angioplasty was successful;

in one patient the final lumen achieved by a 2.1 mm probe was large enough to not require additional balloon dilatation. Chan et al. [8] found that, due to confining the high temperatures to a tiny thermal band around the probe, it was not necessary to apply continuous forward and backward motion to cool the device and to avoid adherence of the probe to the vessel wall, as is described for the original hot-tip laser-probes.

Radiofrequency angioplasty

Currently two types of radiofrequency angioplasty devices are used in clinical studies. Grundfest et al. [27] described a hot-tip system driven by radiofrequency energy instead of laser. In the completely insulated device the ratiofrequency energy is used indirectly for heating the metal tip of the probe, but there is no direct-current flow through the atherosclerotic tissue. With this indirect radiofrequency thermal angioplasty device Grundfest et al. [27] achieved results similar to the hot-tip laserprobe in femoral arteries, but it has not yet been used in coronary vessels.

Our group has used direct radiofrequency angioplasty in a limited number of coronary arteries [34, 35]. By this technique, the radiofrequency current is delivered directly onto the atherosclerotic tissue by a monopolar catheter electrode. The catheter is completely insulated with the exception of a small electrode ring at the front surface of tip. The radiofrequency current heats the plaque directly adjacent to the electrode. Due to the small surface area of the ring-shaped electrode, a high-power, dense electric field is yielded only very close to the electrode, which is thought to minimize thermal damage to the free vascular wall and to minimize thrombus formation within the blood. Radiofrequency angioplasty was used in thirteen patients in the coronary arteries with a success rate of 77% (stenosis reduction > 20%). In four patients additional balloon dilatation was required because stenosis reduction was inadequate. Vessel occlusion occurred in one patient after radiofrequency application; this was successfully treated by balloon dilatation (Table 6).

Laserballoon angioplasty

In laser balloon angioplasty, the arterial wall surrounding an inflated balloon is heated with laser energy to a tissue subvaporization threshold. The concept of laser balloon angioplasty is to create a large, smooth lumen, which is less thrombogenetic, and to avoid initimal dissections and recoil of the elastic parts of the arterial wall as potential causes of complications following balloon dilatation. In experimental studies it has been shown that heating of the vascular wall results in a plaque-arterial wall tissue fusion and reduction of viscoelastic recoil (detailed discussion in [71]). Therefore, laser balloon angioplasty is thought to be an adjunct to balloon dilatation, resulting in a kind of "endogenous stent" for prevention of acute occlusion and restenosis.

Spears et al. [72] recently reported on 65 patients, in whom laser balloon angioplasty could be successfully performed in 62 patients after elective PTCA, resulting in a significant increase of residual stenosis diameter from 1.7 ± 0.6 mm after PTCA to 2.3 ± 0.3 mm after additional laser balloon treatment. There were three acute closures that could be reopened and fixed by balloon angioplasty. Complications of laser balloon angioplasty, as reported by Spears during oral presentation, were one dissection, one embolus, one coronary aneurysma, and ventricular fibrillation in two patients, resulting in an overall complication rate of 8% (Table 6). Especially ventricular fibrillation caused by heating of the arterial wall seems to be a potential harmful complication, since from the NHBLI registry it is known that ventricular fibrillation during balloon dilatation is associated with a 14% mortality and a 48% incidence of nonfatal infarction [33]. Knudtson et al. [44] reported a prospective trial with laser balloon angioplasty in 10 patients following balloon recanalization of occluded coronary arteries as compared to 10 patients receiving laser balloon angioplasty after elective PTCA of stenosed vessels. Although excellent results were found at 48 h after laser balloon angioplasty, without difference in the pot-PTCA diameter, restenosis after 4 months occurred in 4/10 patients with previously occluded vessels, and in 2/10 patients with balloon laserangioplasty of stenosed coronary arteries. Therefore, with the present technology the problem of late restenosis seems not to have been solved by laser balloon angioplasty.

Coronary Atherectomy

At present, mainly two types of coronary atherectomy devices are used in clinical studies.

Simpson atherectomy catheter

The Simpson atherectomy catheter, which has been previously used in several studies in peripheral arteries, consists of a metal housing that incorporates a battery-powered and operator-controlled rotary knife (2000 rpm) [68]. After placement of the atherectomy catheter within the coronary lesion, the rotary knife can be moved within the metal housing to slice off plaque material projecting into the housing from the open side. Cut off plaque material will be stored in the tip of the housing and can be analyzed after removal of the catheter. Therefore, beside its therapeutic value, the Simpson atherectomy device allows a selective percutaneous biopsy of atheromatous tissue for further histologic analysis and cell culture [5, 11, 60].

Clinical experience in more than 500 patients is available with the Simpson atherectomy device (Table 7). Pinkerton et al. [57] reported a 90% success rate with the treatment of

Table 7. Coronary atherectomy.

Author	Method	Pat. No.	Lesion No	Success Rate	Compli- cation	Death	AMI	CABG	Other
Pinkerton 1989	Simpson	394	440	90%	8%	2	3	20 5%	2 emboli 5 side br. occlusion
Vlietstra 1989	Simpson	480	534	88%	18%	3	23 5%	21 4,4%	1 stroke 11 emboli 1 perforation
Fourier 1989	Fast Rotation	12	12	83%	0%	0	0	0	3 AV-block
Ginsburg 1989	Fast Rotation	40	40	?	15%	0	5	1	12 spasm (30%)
O'Neill 1989	Fast Rotation	30	30	97%	20%	0	5	1	20% no- reflow

440 lesions of 394 patients. In this study the complication rate was 8%, including 20 emergency treatments with bypass grafting, two deaths, three myocardial infarctions, two emboli, and five side branch occlusions. Recently, Vlietstra et al. [76] gave a detailed report about the complications in a large multicenter trial in which directional atherectomy was applied in 534 lesions of 480 patients with a success rate of 88%. Complications occurred in 86/480 (18%) of patients. Vessel occlusion was seen in 4.7%, branch vessel occlusion in 4.0%, coronary embolism in 2.3%, spasm in 1.6%, coronary dissection by the guide catheter in 0.6%, perforation in one patient (0.2%), ventricular fibrillation in 1.5%, significant vascular complications in 1.2%, stroke in one patient (0.2%), and device complications in 0.8%. These events led to emergency bypass surgery in 4.4% and to emergency balloon dilatation in 2.0%. Myocardial infarction occurred in 3 patients (4.8%), including three Q-wave infarctions; three ptients (0.6%) died. Overall there was a 5.8% rate of major events such as deaths, Q-wave infarction, emergency surgery, and stroke.

Restenosis rate after directional coronary atherectomy is 38% in native coronary arteries and 55% in venous grafts, which is quite similar to the results of balloon dilatation [70].

High-speed rotational angioplasty

This technique uses the abrasive effect of a high-speed rotating burr (180 000 rpm) for removal of atherosclerotic tissue instead of extracting it as is done by the Simpson atherectomy device. After successful experimental and peripheral studies [29, 2], the Rotablator has recently been used in the coronary arteries, as well. In the first report, Fourrier et al. [20] achieved a stenosis reduction of > 20% in 10/12 (83%) coronary lesions of 2 patients. In five patients residual stenosis exceeded 50% (60 ± 3%) and required additional balloon dilatation; in the other five patients high-speed rotational angioplasty alone was sufficient (mean stenosis reduction from 73% to 46%). Fourier et al. [20] did not observe any acute complications with the exception of a transient atrioventricular block in three patients without subsequent ECG changes or rise of serum creatine kinase. The development of a transient AV-block, which has been suggested to be caused by rotation-induced vibration, seems to be a specific complication of high-speed rotational angioplasty and has also been reported by other investigators [18].

Ginsburg et al. [23] reported on 40 patients, in whom rotational atherectomy achieved an increase of the mean arterial diameter from 1.6 ± 0.2 mm to 2.1 ± 0.1 mm without complementary balloon dilatation. The complication rate was relatively high in that study, including transient spasm in 30%, creatine kinase elevation in 20%, ventricular stunning in 12.5%, and emergency bypass surgery in one patient (2.5%), but there was no death and no Q-wave infarction.

O'Neill et al. [55] reported a 97% success rate of high-speed rotational angioplasty in 30 patients, in whom residual stenosis was less than 50% without additional balloon dilatation. Also in that study, the rate of minor complications was relatively high, including creatine kinase increase in 16%, transient cessation of flow in 20%, and emergency surgery in one patient (3%). Follow-up angiography after 6 months revealed a restenosis rate of 44%, which is at least equal to that of balloon dilatation.

References

1. Abela GS, Seeger JM, Barbieri E, Fronzini D, Fenech A, Pepine CJ, Conti CR (1986) Laser angioplasty with angioscopic guidance in humans. J Am Coll Cardiol 8:184–192
2. Ahn SS, Auth DC, Marcus DR, Moore WS (1988) Removl of focal atheromatous lesions by angioscopically guided high-speed rotary atherectomy. J Vasc Surg 7:292–299

3. Alford WC, Stoney WS, Page HL, Burrus GR, Glassford DM, Petracek MR, Thomas CS (1982) Surgical procedures after percutaneous transluminal coronary angioplasty. South Med J 75:1556–1558
4. Aueron F, Gruentzig A (1984) Distal embolization of a coronary bypass graft atheroma during percutaneous transluminal coronary angioplasty. Am J. Cardiol 53:953–954
5. Bauriedel G, Dartsch PC, Voisard R, Roth D, Simpson JB, Höfling B, Betz E (1989) Selective percutaneous biops of atheromatous plaque tissue for cell culture. Basic Res Cardiol 84:326–331
6. Buchwald A, Werner GS, Unterberg C, Voth E, Figulla HR, Wiegand V (1989) Excimer-Laser-Koronarangioplastie hochgradiger Stenosen und chronischer Okklusionen. Z Kardiol 78: 714–718
7. Cairns JA, Collins R, Fuster V, Passamani ER (1989) Coronary thrombolysis. Chest 95:73S–87S
8. Chan MC, Lee G, Jing-Xuan G, Mao JU, Chen F, Yan W, Xie D, Rink DL, Argenal AJ, Mason DT (1989) Percutaneous coronary laser angioplasty using quick short bursts of laser thermal energy for chronic total occlusions. Am J Cardiol 64:940–942
9. Choy DSJ, Stertzer SH, Myler RK, Marco J, Fournial G (1984) Human coronary laser recanalization. Clin Cardiol 7:377–381
10. Côté G, Stertzer SH, Mylr RK, Bonan R, Andrus WS, Roth L, Lane J, Dumont M, Maden M, Hidalgo BO (1989) Early clinical experience with percutaneous transluminal argon laser coronary angioplasty. J Am Coll Cardiol 13:61A (abstr.)
11. Dartsch PC, Voisard R, Bauriedel G, Höfling B, Betz E (1990) Growth characteristics and cytosceletal organisation of cultered smooth muscle cells from primary and restenosed lesions Arteriosclerosis 10:62–75
12. Detre K, Holubkov R, Kelsey S, Cowley M, Kent K, Williams D, Myler R, Faxon D, Holmes Jr D, Bourassa M, Block P, Gosselin A, Bentivoglio L, Leatherman L, Dorros G, King III S, Galichia J, Al-Bassam M, Leon M, Robertson T, Passamani E (1988) Percutaneous transluminal coronary angioplasty in 1985–1986 and 1977–1981. The National Heart, Lung, and Blood Institute Registry. N Engl J Med 138: 265–270
13. Detre K, Holubkov R, Kelsey S, Bourassa M, Williams D, Holmes Jr D, Dorros G, Faxon D, Myler R, Kent K, Cowley M, Cannon R, Robertson T (1989) One-year follow-up results of the 1985–1986 National Heart, Lung, and Blood Institute's Percutaneous transluminal coronary angioplasty registry. Circulation 80:421–428
14. Dorros G, Lewin RF, Mathiak LM, Johnson WD, Brenowitz J, Schmahl T, Tector A (1988) Percutaneous transluminal coronary angioplasty in patients with two or more previous coronary artery bypass grafting operations. Am J Cardiol 61:1243–1247
15. Douglas JS Jr, Gruentzig AR, King SB III, Hollman J, Ischingr T, Meier B, Carver JM, Jones EL, Waller JL, Bone DK, Gyuton R (1983) Percutaneous transluminal coronary angioplasty in patients with prior coronary bypass surgery. J Am Coll Cardiol 2: 745–754
16. Ellis SG, Roubin GS, King SB, Douglas JS, Shaw RE, Stertzer SH, Myler RK (1988) In-hospital cardiac mortality after acute closure after coronary angioplasty: Analysis of risk factors from 8,207 procedures. J Am Coll Cardiol 11:211–216
17. Ellis SG, O'Neill WW, Bates ER, Walton JA, Nabel EG, Werns SW, Topol EJ (1989) Implications for patient triage from survival and left ventricular functional recovery analyses in 500 patients treated with coronary angioplasty for acute myocardial infarction. J Am Coll Cardiol 13:1251–1259
18. Erbel R, Dietz U, Mixdorf U, Haude M, Rupprecht HJ, Auth D, Meyer J (1989) Koronare Hochfrquenz-Rotations-Arteiektomie. Z Kardiol 78 (Suppl 1): 21 (abstr.)
19. Foschi AE, Zapala CA (1989) Direct argon laser irradiation of high-grade stenoses and total occlusions in native human coronary arteries and bypass grafts: Initial clinical experience. J Am Coli Cardiol 13: 60A (abstr.)
20. Fourrier JL, Bertrand ME, Auth DC, Lablanche JM, Gommeaux A, Brunetaud JM (1989) Percutaneous coronary rotational angioplasty in Humans: Preliminary report. J Am Coll Cardiol 14:1278–1282
21. Garrison BJ, Srinivasan R (1984) Microscopic model for the ablative photodecomposition of polymers by far ultraviolet radiation (193 nm). Appl Phys Lett 44:849–851
22. Gaul G, Hollman J, Simpfendorfr C, Franco I (1989) Acute occlusion in multiple lesion coronary angioplasty: Frequency and management. J. Am Coll Cardiol 13:283–288
23. Ginsburg R, Wexler L, Mitchell RS, Profitt D (1985) Percutaneous transluminal laser angioplasty for treatment of peripheral vascular disease: clinical experience with sixteen patients
24. Ginsburg R, Teirstein PS, Warth DC, Haw N, Jenkins NS, McCowan LC (1989) Percutaneous transluminal coronary rotational atheroblation: Clinical experience in 40 patients. Circulation 80:II–584 (abstr.)
25. Grüntzig AR, Senning A, Siegenthaler WE (1970) Nonopertive dilation of coronary–artery stenosis: percutaneous transluminal coronary angioplasty. N Engl J Med 301:61–68
26. Grundfest WS, Litvack IF, Goldenberg T, Shermann T, Morgenstern L, Carroll R, Fishbein M,

Forrester J, Margitan J, McDermid S (1985) Pulsed ultraviolet lasers and the potential for safe laser angioplasty. Am J Surg 150:220–226

27. Grundfest W, Litvack F, Hickey A, Adler L, Foran R, Lewin P, Segalowitz J, Hestrin L, Forrester J (1989) Radiofrequency thermal angioplasty for the treatment of peripheral vascular occlusiove disease: Preliminary results of a clinical trial. J Am Coll Cardiol 13:14A (abstr.)

28. Hamad N, Pichard A, Lyle HRP, Lindsay J (1988) Results of percutaneous transluminal coronary angioplasty by multiple, relatively low frequency operators: 1986–1987 experience. Am J Cardiol 61:1229–1231

29. Hansen DD, Auth DC, Vrocko R, Ritchie JL (1988) Rotational atherectomy in atherosclerotic rabbit iliac arteries. Am Heart J 115:160–165

30. Harston WE, Tilley S, Rodeheffer R, Formann MB, Perry JM (1986) Safety and success of the beginning percutaneous transluminal coronary angioplasty program using the sterrable guidewire system. Am J Cardiol 57:7K–10K

31. Higgins CB (1988) Coronary angiography: A decade of advances. Am J Cardiol 62: 7K–10K

32. Hollman J, Gruentzig AR, Douglas JS Jr, King SB, Ischinger T, Meier B (1983) Acute occlusion after percutaneous transluminal coronary angioplasty – a new approach. Circulation 68:725–732

33. Holmes DR, Holubkov R, Vlietstra RE, Kelsey SF, Reeder GS, Dorros G, Williams DO, Cowley MJ, Faxon DP, Kent KM, Bentivoglio LG, Detre K (1988) Comparison of complications during percutaneous transluminal coronary angioplasty from 1977 to 1981 and from 1985 to 1986: The National Heart, Lung, and Blood Institute Percutaneous Transluminal Coronary Angioplasty Registry. J. Am Coll Cardiol 12:149–155

34. Hombach V, Höher M, Höpp HW, Kochs M, Eggeling T, Osypka P, Hilger HH (1988) Erste klinische Erfahrungen mit der Hochfrequenzangioplastie bei Patienten mit koronarer Herzkrankheit. Dtsch Med Wschr 113, 801–805

35. Hombach V, Höher M, Kochs M, Wieshammer S, Haerer W, Eggeling T, Schmidt A, Höpp HW, Hilger HH (1989) Radiofrequency coronary angioplasty in patients with coronary artery disease – a new method for treatment of coronary artery stenoses. In: Höfling B, v Pölnitz A (eds): Interventional cardiology and angiology. Steinkopff Verlag, Darmstadt, 163–168

36. Isley CDJ, Ablett MD (1986) Percutaneous transluminal coronary angioplasty in multilesion disease: complete versus incomplete revascularization. Tex Heart Inst J 13:371–376

37. Jacob AS, Pichard AD, Ohnmacht SD, Lindsay J (1986) Results of percutaneous transluminal coronary angioplasty by multiple relatively low frequency operators. Am J Cardiol 57: 713–716

38. James TN (1965) Anatomy of the coronary arteries in health and disease. Circulation 32:1020–1029

39. Kaltenbach M, Kober G, Scherer D, Vallbracht C (1985) Recurrence rate after successful coronary angioplasty. Eur Heart J 6:276–281

40. Karsch KR, Haase KK, Mauser M, Ickrath O, Voelker W, Duda S, Seipel L (1989) Perkutane transluminale koronare Excimer-Laserangioplastie. Dtsch Med Wschr 114:1183–1187

41. Keogh B, Crea F, Bull T, Blackie S, Taylor KM (1988) An in vitro study to assess the risk of embolism following lasing human coronary atherosclerotic plaque with metal-capped optical fibers. Eur Heart J 9 (Suppl 1): 235 (abstr.)

42. Keogh B, Crea F, Pashazadeh M, Blackie RAS, Taylor KM (1988) Lasing in blood with metal-capped optical fibres: The potential hazard of distal thrombembolism. Eur Heart J 9 (Suppl 1): 235 (abstr.)

43. King SB (1988) Percutaneous transluminal coronary angioplasty: The second decade. Am J Cardiol 62:2K–6K

44. Knudtson ML, Spindler BM, Traboulsi M, Spears JR (1989) Coronary laser balloon angioplasty in chronic total occlusion provides excellent short-term results. Circulation 80:II–476 (abstr.)

45. Lee G, Ikeda RM, Kozina J, Mason DT (1981) Laser-dissolution of coronary atherosclerotic obstruction. Am Heart J 102:1074–1075

46. Linnemeier TJ, Cumberland DC, Rothbaum DA, Landin RJ, Ball MW (1989) Human percutaneous laser-assisted coronary angioplasty: Efforts to reduct spasm and thrombosis. J Am Coll Cardiol 13: 61A (abstr.)

47. Litvack F, Grundfest WS, Goldenberg T (1988) Pulsed laser angioplasty: wavelength power and energy dependencies relevant to clinical application

48. Litvack F, Grundfest WS, Goldenberg T, Laudenslager J, Forrester JS (1989) Percutaneous excimer laser angioplasty of aortocoronary saphenous vein grafts. J Am Coll Cardiol 14: 803–808

49. Margolis JR, Litvack F, Grundfest W, Eigler N, Goldenberg T, Laudenslager J, Tsoi D, Wong S, Segalowitz J, Hestrin L, Rothbaum D, Linnemeier T, Helfant R, Forrester J (1989) Excimer laser coronary angioplasty: Results of a multicenter study. Circulation 80:II–477 (abstr.)

50. Meier B (1987) Coronary angioplasty. Grune & Stratton Inc., Orlando

51. Meier B, King SB, Gruentzig AR, Douglas JS, Hollman J, Ischinger T, Galan K, Tankersley R (1984) Repeat coronary angioplasty. J. Am Coll Cardiol 4:463–466

52. Meier B, Gruentzig A, King S, Douglas J, Hollman J, Ischinger T, Galan K (1984) Higher balloon dilatation pressure in coronry angioplasty. Am Heart J 107:619–62
53. Myler RK, Topol EJ, Shaw RE, Stertzer SH, Clark DA, Fishman J, Murphy MC (1987) Multiple vessel coronary angioplasty: classification, results and patterns of restenosis in 494 consecutive patients. Cathet Cardiovasc Diagn 13:1–15
54. O'Keefe JH Jr, Rutherford BD, McConahay DR, Ligon RW, Johnson WL, Giogi LV, Crockett JE, McCallister BD, Conn RD, Gura GM, Good TH, Steinhaus DM, Bateman TM, Shimshak TM, Hartzler GO (1989) Early and late results of coronary angioplasty without antecedent therombolytic therapy for acute myocardial infarction. Am J Cardiol 64:221–1230
55. O'Neill WW, Friedman HZ, Cragg D, Strzelecki MR, Gangadharan V, Levine AB, Ramos RG (1989) Initial clinical experience and early follow-up of patients undergoing mechanical rotary endarterectomy. Circulation 80:II–584 (abstr.)
56. Oomen A, Tuntelder JR, Velema E, Verdaasdonk RM, Rienks R, Borst C (1988) Laser-heated metal probe recanalisation of aortic stenosis in the rabbit: embolisation and wall damage. Eur Heart J 9 (Suppl 1): 235 (abstr.)
57. Pinkerton C, Simpson J, Selmon M, Robertson G, Hinohara T, Hollman J, Baim D (1989) Percutaneous coronary atherectomy: Early experiences of multicenter trial. J Am Coll Cardiol 13: 108A (abstr.)
58. Reeder GS, Breshnahan JF, Holmes DR Jr, Mock MB, Orszulak TA, Smith HC, Vlietstra RE (1986) Angioplasty for aortocoronary bypass graft stenosis. Mayo Clin Proc 61:14–19
59. Roubin GS, Douglas Jr JS, King III SB, Lin S, Hutchison N, Thomas RG, Gruentzig AR (1988) Influence of balloon size on initial success, acute complications, and restenosis after percutaneous transluminal coronary angioplasty. A prospective randomized study. Circulation 78:557–565
60. Safian RD, Gelbfish JS, Erny RE, Schnitt S, Baim DS (1989) Histologic findings of coronary atherectomy. Circulation 80:II–583 (abstr.)
61. Sanborn TA, Faxon DP, Haudenschild CC, Ryan TJ (1985) Experimental angioplasty: Circumferential distribution of laser thermal energy with a laser probe. J. Am Coll Cardiol 5:934–938
62. Sanborn TA, Haudenschild CC, Faxon DP, Garber GR, Ryan TJ (1987) Angiographic and histologic consequences of laser thermal angioplasty: Comparison with balloon angioplasty. Circulation 75:281–286
63. Sanborn TA, Cumberland DC (1989) Laserprobe. In: Isner JM, Clarke RH (eds): Cardiovascular laser therapy. Raven Press, New York. 149–162
64. Schmitz HJ, Von Essen R, Meyer J, Effert S (1984) The role of balloon size for acute and late angiographic results in coronary angiography. Circultion 70 (suppl II): II–295 (abstr.)
65. Schömig A, Brachmann J, Müller—Bühl U, Scheidt D, Wilhelm C, Kübler W (1989) Klinische Anwendung eines Argon-Laser-Systems bei peripheren and coronaren Arterienverschlüssen. Z Kardiol 78 (Suppl 1): 21 (abstr.)
66. Simoons ML, Arnold AE, Betriu A, de Bono DP, Col J, Dougherty FC, von Essen R, Lambertz H, Lubsen J, Meier B (1988) Thrombolysis with tissue plasminogen activator in acute myocardial infarction: no additional benefit from immediate percutaneous coronary angioplasty. Lancet: 197–202
67. Simpfendorfer C, Belardi J, Bellamy G, Galan K, Franco I, Hollman J (1987) Frequency, management, and follow-up of patients with acute coronary occlusion after percutaneous transluminal coronaiy angioplasty. Am J Cardiol 59.267–259
68. Simpson JB, Selmon MR, Robertson GC, Cipriano PR, Hayden WG, Johnson DE, Fogarty TJ (1988) Transluminal atherectomy for occlusive peripheral vascular disease. Am J Cardiol 61:93G–101G
69. Simpson JB, Baim DS, Robert EW, Harrison DC (1982) A new catheter system for coronary angioplasty. Am J Cardiol 49:1216–1222
70. Simpson JB, Robertson GC, Selmon MR, Sipperly E, Braden LJ, Hinohara T (1989) Restenosis following successful directional coronary atherectomy. Circulation 80:II–582
71. Spears JR (1989) Sealing. In: Isner JM, Clarke RH (eds): Cardiovascular laser therapy. Raven Press, New York, 177–199
72. Spears JR, Dear WE, Safian RD, Sinclair IN, Plokker HWM, Aldridge H, Knudtson ML, Sigwart U, Rickards AF (1989) Laser balloon angioplasty: Angiographic results of a multicenter trial. Circulation 80:II–476 (abstr.)
73. TIMI Study Group (1989) Comparison of invasive and conservative strategies after treatment with intravenous tissue plasminogen activator in acute myocardial infarction. New Engl J Med 320:618–627
74. Teirstein PS, Hoover CA, Ligon RW, Giorgi LV, Rutherford BD, McConahay DR, Johnson WL, Hartzler GO (1989) Repeat coronary angioplasty: Efficacy of a third angioplasty for a secon restenosis. J Am Coll Cardiol 13:291–296
75. Topol EJ, Califf RM, George BS, Kereiakes DH, Abbottsmith CW, Candela RJ, Lee KL, Pitt B, Stack

RS, O'Neill WW (1987) A randomized trial of immediate versus delayed elective angioplasty after intravenous tissue plasminogen activator in acute myocardial infarction. N Engl J Med 317:581–588
76. Vlietstra RE, Abbotsmith CW, Douglas JS, Hollman JL, Muller D, Safian R, Selmon MR (1989) Complications with directional coronary atherectomy. Experience at eight centers. Circulation 80 (Suppl II), II–582 (abstr.)
77. Williams DO, Grüntzig AR, Kent KM, Detre KM, Kelsey SF, to T (1984) Efficacy of repeat percutaneous transluminal coronary angioplasty for coronary restenosis. Am J Cardiol 53:32C–35C.

Author's address
Dr. Martin Höher
University Ulm
Department of Cardiology-Pneumonology-Angiology
Robert-Koch-Str. 8
7900 Ulm, FRG

Management of Complications

Emergency CABG - Surgery after PTCA: Complications in 1420 Cases of Angioplasty, with Consideration of Coronary Anatomy, Management, and Outcome

E. Frantz, J. Krülls-Münch, H. Oswald, E. Fleck

German Heart Institute, Berlin, FRG

Introduction

Since the number of different techniques of invasive cardiologic treatment has increased, it is necessary to define indications and contraindications of those techniques, where the largest amount of experience has been gathered. In order to identify the predictors for early unfavorable outcome of the procedure, we retrospectively analyzed all coronary angioplasty procedures performed in our clinic. Attention was also directed on the coronary anatomy of the treated patients, and on the post-complication management and outcome of complicated procedures.

Evaluated samples

From April 1986 to December 1989 in the German Heart Institute, Berlin, 1420 patients underwent percutaneous transluminal coronary anagioplasty (PTCA).

Five of these patients underwent angioplasty with preexisting cardiogenic shock after acute myocardial infarction. Since particularities in those cases are rather distinct to elective treatment, those cases were evaluated separately in the present study. Three of these patients (who were not acceptable for CABG-surgery because of their coronary anatomy) died; two had undergone emergency bypass surgery.

Of the 1420 cases of PTCA presented in this paper, 1164 patients (= 82%) were men, 256 (18%) were women.

Eighteen of these 1420 patients (1.27%) were eligible for emergency coronary-artery-bypass grafting because of in-lab complications. In the following, this subset is analyzed.

Mean age of these 18 patients (15 male, 3 female) was 58.9 years (+/- 9.0), mean LV-ejection fraction was 56.3 +/- 7.2%. Vessel involvement in these patients was distributed as shown in Table 1.

Table 1. Evaluated sample: vessel involvement.

	n =
3-Vessel disease	1
2-Vessel disease	8
1-Vessel disease	7
1-Vessel disease + LMCA-Plaque	2
	18

Procedures

In all but one patient, balloon inflations could be performed, and stenosis dilation was primarily successful. In one patient, the coronary artery was perforated by the attempt to open the chronically occluded vessel. Mean number of balloon inflations was 6.4 +/- 3.6, mean duration was 261 +/- 157 s. Inflations as part of the elective treatment action cannot be separated from inflations as part of the complication-handling in every patient.

In 11 patients, one-vessel/one-stenosis dilation was intended; in five patients, two vessels with one stenosis in each vessel was targeted; in two patients a multilesion-dilation in one vessel was intended. In total, 26 stenoses were targareted. The localization and severity of these stenoses are noted in Tables 2–4.

According to frequently used and well defined characteristics of coronary artery stenoses, the morphology of coronary arteries was described as noted in Table 4.

Table 2. Localization of target stenoses.

Vessel	Prox.	Med.	Dist.	1st Branch	2nd Branch	Total
LAD	8	8	3	1	–	20
LCX	1	–	1	3	–	5
RCA	–	1	–	–	–	1
Stenoses						26

Patients, n = 18

Table 3. Severity of stenoses (pre-PTCA).

Occluded (= 100%)	1
99%	1
90%	19
75%	4
< 75%	1
Stenoses	26

Patients, n = 18

Table 4. Stenosis morphology characteristics (pre-PTCA).

Branch point	12
Length > 2 lumen diameters	11
Other stenosis - proximal	6
Excentricity	5
Ulcus/rough lumen	3
Abrupt proximal face	3
Thrombus	2
Other stenosis - distal	2
Diffuse disease	1
Delayed dye flow	1

n = 18 patients, 26 stenoses

Balloon size

Since one of the essentials of the procedure and of its risk for unfavorable outcome is the question of an adequate balloon size, in all cases a visual retrospective analysis was

Table 5. Balloon/vessel cross-section relation.

Balloon size	Vessel diameter Proximal stenosis (mm)	Vessel diameter Distal stenosis (mm)	Balloon cross-section (mm)
Appropriate	3,1 +/- 0,62	2,6 +/- 0,35	2,7 +/- 0,24
Undersized	3,4 +/- 0,35	3,1 +/- 0,25	2,5 +/- 0,29

Patients, n = 12

undertaken. The balloon was not angiographically documented in all cases, but balloon size of 12/18 patients could be evaluated.

Compared to vessel cross-section (proximal and distal to the attacked stenosis), in six cases the balloon seemed to be of appropriate size, in six cases it was undersized; no instance of an oversized balloon could be identified. These data are given in detail in Table 5.

Complications/outcome

The outcome of the 1420 angioplasty-procedures is given in Fig. 1. Regarding the 18 patients in whom emergency CABG-surgery became necessary, severity of stenoses and charasteristics of coronary morphology *post-PTCA* are given in Tables 6–8.

Periprocedural myocardial infarction

Of the 14 patients who survived emergency bypass surgery after PTCA, six showed either ECG or chemical signs of periopertaive myocardial infarction.

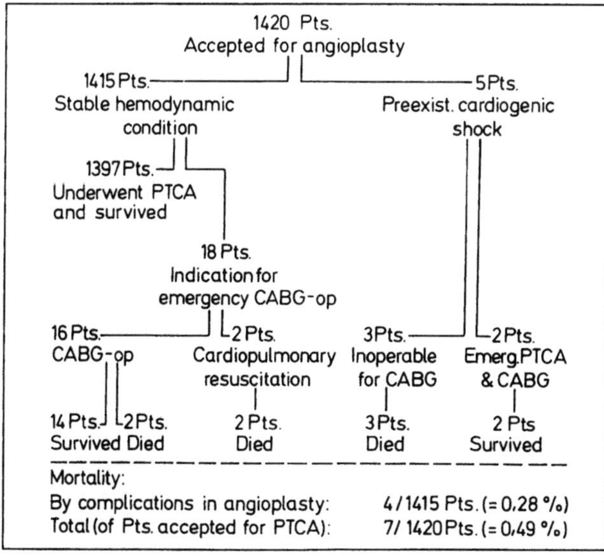

Fig. 1. Outcome of the 1420 angioplasty-procedures.

Table 6. Lumen reduction in target stenoses (post-PTCA).

Occluded (= 100%)	16
99%	3
90%	3
75%	3
< 75%	3
Stenoses	26

Patients, n = 18

Table 7. Stenosis morphology characteristics (post-PTCA).

Intimal tear/dissesction	16
Length > 2 lumen diameters	6
Ulcus/rough lumen	3
Branch point	2
Thrombus	1
Vessel perforation	1
Other stenosis - proximal	1
Other stenosis - distal	1
Diffuse disease	1
Delayed dye flow	1
Excentricity	–
Abrupt proximal face	–
Stenoses, total	26

Patients, n = 18

Table 8. Balloon/vessel cross-section relation; comparison of appropriate vs undersized balloons used.

Post-PTCA stenosis Morphology/Quantity	Appropriate balloon size n = 6 pts.	Balloon undersized n = 6 pts.
Dilated vessel occluded	5	4
Dissection	6	6
Diss. length > 2 lumen diameter	2	2
Vessel branch occluded	2	2
Dilated stenosis < 90%	1	2

For the cases in which baloon-size evaluation was possible, coronary morphology was compared between the groups with adequate and undersized balloon diameters. Table 8 shows the incidences of different morphologic characteristics.

Complication management

The five patients with pre-existing cardiogenic shock had been accepted for PTCA because of unstable angina. In three of them (all having undergone CABG years before) prior coronary angiography had revealed no possibility for successful repeat bypass grafting. Because of three-vessel-disease with total or subtotal multilesion pattern in all vessels, successful angioplasty could not be performed.

In the remaining two patients with pre-existing cardiogenic shock successful emergency PTCA and immediate consecutive surgical revascularization were performed.

As coronary angioplasty in this clinic is performed in a cath-lab, which is a fully-equipped operating theater, there was only a minimal time from diagnosis of complication, finding the indication of emergency bypass surgery to beginning of surgical intervention. In none of the reported cases was this more than 60 min. Six of the 18 patients had an autoperfusion catheter implanted for bridging the time until definite revascularization could be achieved.

In two of the 18 patients with angioplasty-related complications, immediate cardio-pulmonary resuscitation was necessary:

One patient, male, 79 years, suffering from unstable angina with a 99% LAD-stenosis, underwent PTCA because of inoperable situs after pericarditis constrictiva and pericardectomy. Twenty min after angioplasty of LAD a large dissection of LAD and LMCA occurred; consequently, LMCA was occluded. Ventricular fibrillation led to immediate breakdown of circulation and cardiopulmonary resuscitation was unsuccessful. The second patient, female, 68 years, had undergone PTCA 24 h before the acute event: sudden cardiogenic shock occurred, coronary thrombosis was angiographically documented, and cardiopulmonary resuscitation was unsuccessful. In both patients, extracorporal circulation could not be established.

The other 16/18 patients with indication for emergency bypass-surgery exhibited stable circulation pre-operatively.

Of the patients with emergency CABG-indication, two patients died intraoperatively because of stunned myocardium at the end of extracorporal circulation. In both patients, stable hemodynamic conditions had been established after angioplasty complication and before surigical intervention. Stunned myocardium occurred in myocardial area not being supplied by angioplasty-target vessels.

Literature review/discussion

Complication incidence

Of the 3079 patients enrolled in the original NHLBI PTCA registry, 1978–1981, 29 patients died, mortaility rate of 0.29%. In 202 patients (6.4%) emergency bypass surgery was necessary; 13 patients died intraoperatively. In 44.8% of the patients who died, emergency surgery had been undertaken [1,3,7,8].

Newer figures indicate that in approximately 4% of PTCA-patients abrupt vessel closure occurs during the first 30 min after angioplasty. In half of those vessels this is due to immediate re-dilatation, leaving approximately 2.5% of total PTCA procedures to instead result in emergency CABG.

Comparison of the figures in the present series with NHLBI PTCA-registry figures is shown in Table 9.

Mortality rates in all three series are quite comparable, showing that improvement in equipment and experience may be balanced by acceptance of patients at higher risk for PTCA in all three periods. However, necessity for emergency surgical intervention con-

Table 9. Comparison of present series with NHLBI PTCA registry.

Outcome		NHLBI PTCA registry 1978–1981	NHLBI PTCA registry 1985–1986	This series 1986–1989
Patients	n =	3079	1801	1415
Death	n/%)	29/0.29	18/1.0	4/0.28
Emergency CABG	(n/%)	202/6.4	63/3.5	18/1.27

Table 10. Influencing criteria.

	Prior studies	Pts. total	Pts. with complication	Pts. in studies with significant influence of criterium for complications		Present study (18 pts. with emerg. CABG after PTCA complication; 26 stenoses)
	No.	n	%	n /	%	No. of stenoses
Excentricity	5	8367	9.0	8127	97.1	5
Branch point	3	5312	5.7	5072	95.4	12
Bend point	2	4712	5.3	4472	94.9	–
Thrombus	2	4712	5.3	4472	94.9	2
Dissection	4	5308	4.8	4782	90.1	3
Length of stenosis	3	5238	5.3	4472	85.4	11

tinuously decreases, especially since steerable guidewire devices allow immediate repeat re-dilatation.

Coronary anatomy

We have reviewed seven studies [2,4,5,6,9–11] from 1983 to 1989 that report on coronary morphology as predictor of acute vessel closure after PTCA. Significant influence on the risk of acute PTCA complications was found for the criteria shown in Table 10.

The following criteria did not prove significant influence on complication risks in any prior study (the number of stenoses fulfilling the criterion in the present study, is given (in parenthesis)): other stenosis in the same vessel (8), stenosis located in LAD (20), calcification in stenosis pressure gradient before PTCA, ulceration (3), and abrupt proximal stenosis face (3).

Conclusions

This review of 1420 cases accepted for PTCA shows a decreased incidence of in-lab complications, compared to the risk-ratio in the NHLBI series of two periods in the 1980s. This might be an effect of improved technical equipment, as well as increased clinical experience. Since more patients with complex coronary anatomy are accepted for angioplasty nowadays, who are at greater risk for unsuccessful outcome, mortality has not yet been markedly reduced. However, contemporary angioplasty techniques provide a possibility of revascularization, even for those patients who are not eligible for surgical intervention.

Despite rapid surgical intervention, some of the patients surviving emergency CABG-operation suffered from perioperative myocardial infarction. Thus, despite the decreasing incidence of in-lab complications after PTCA, it is noteworthy that every complication bears a considerable risk for the patient.

In order to identify the circumstances that led to early angioplasty complications in this series, coronary anatomy was considered. Especially, stenoses at branch points, excentric stenoses, those with rough surface and of certain length were found to be at risk for the occurrence of acute vessel occlusion in case of large dissection after angioplasty.

In this study, nearly all patients (due to emergency CABG-operation after PTCA) suffered from one- or two-vessel coronary artery disease, showing that risk for in-lab complications is not concentrated in patients with a high-extent of coronary artery disease.

In spite of some cases with PTCA-complications caused by multiple-lesion angio-plasties, no case could be identified in which multiple-vessel intervention was the cause for the complication.

Thus, early complications after PTCA do not emerge from complex CAD vessel involvement or from multilesion treatment procedures, but they are correlated to pre-existing anatomic pecularities of the target lesions.

References

1. Cowley MJ. Dorros G, Kelsey SF, van Raden M, Detre KM. (1984) Acute Coronary Events Associated with PTCA. Am J Cardiol 53, Suppl.C: 12C–16C
2. Cowley MJ, Dorros G, Kelsey SF, van Raden M, Detre KM (1984) Emergency Coronary Bypass Surgery After Coronary Angioplasty: The National Heart, Lung, and Blood Institute's PTCA Registry Experience. Am J Cardiol 53, Suppl.C: 22C–26C
3. Detre K, Holubkov R, Kelsey S, Cowley M, Kent K, Williams D, Myler R, Faxon DP, Holmes D, Bourassa M, Block P, Gosselin A, Bentivoglio L, Leatherman L, Dorros G, King SB III, Galicha J, Al-Bassam M, Leon M, Robertson T, Passamani E (1988) Percutaneous Transluminal Coronary Angioplasty in 1985–1986 and 1977–1981, The National Heart, Lung, and Blood Institute Registry. New England J Med 318: 265–70
4. Ellis S, Roubin GS, King SB III, Douglas JS, Weintraub W, Thomas R, Cox W (1989) Incidence and Predictors of Early Recurrent Ischemia after Successful PTCA for Acute Myocardial Infarction. Am J Card 63: 263–8
5. Ellis S, Roubin GS, King SB III, Douglas JS, Weintraub W, Thomas R, Cox W (1988) Angiographic and Clinical Predictors of acute Closure after Native Vessel Coronary Angioplasty. Circ 77: 372–9
6. Ellis S, Roubin GS, King SB III, Douglas JS, Shaw RE, Stertzer SH. (1988) In-hospital cardiac mortality after acute closure after coronary angioplasty: analysis of risk factors from 8.207 procedures. JACC 11: 211–6
7. Holmes DR, Holubkov R, Vliestra RE, Kelsey SF, Reeder GS, Dorros G, Williams DO, Cowley MJ, Faxon DP, Bentivoglio LG, Detre K (1988) Comparison of Complications During Percutaneous Transluminal Coronary Angioplasty From 1977 to 1981 and From 1985 to 1986: The National Heart, Lung, and Blood Institute Percutaneous Transluminal Coronary Angioplasty Registry. JACC 12: 1149–55
8. Holmes DR, Vliestra RE, Smith HC, Vetrovec GW, Kent KM, Cowley MJ, Faxon DP, Grüntzig AR, Kelsey SF, Detre KM, Van Raden MJ. Mock MB (1984) Restenosis after Percutaneous Transluminal Coronary Angioplasty (PTCA): A Report from the PTCA Registry of the National Heart, Lung, and Blood Institute. Am J Cardio 53, Suppl.C: 77C–81C
9. Meier B, Grüntzig AR, Hollman J, Ischinger T, Bradford J (1983) Does Length or Eccentricity of Coronary stenoses Influence the Outcome of Transluminal Dilatation? Circ 67: 497
10. Meier B, Gruentzig AR, King SB III, Douglas JS, Hollman J. Ischinger T, Aueron F, Galan K (1984) Risk of Side Branch Occlusion During Coronary Angioplasty. Am J Cardio 53: 10–4
11. Simpfendorfer C, Belardi J, Bellamy G, Galan K, Franco I, Hollanm J (1987) Frequency, Management and Follow-Up of Patients with Acute Coronary Occlusions after Percutaneous Transluminal Coronary Angioplasty. Am J Cardio 59: 267–9

Author's address:
Dr. E. Frantz
Klinik für Innere Medizin - Kardiologie
Deutsches Herzzentrum Berlin
Augustenburger Platz 1
1000 Berlin 65, FRG

Acute Coronary Occlusion after PTCA – Management by Redilatation, Perfusion-Catheters, and Stents

A. Buchwald, C. Unterberg, G. S. Werner, U. Tebbe, H. R. Figulla and V. Wiegand

Dept. of Cardiology, University Clinic, Göttingen, FRG

Introduction

Despite continuous improvement in balloon-catheter and guidewire technology, acute coronary occlusion after PTCA occurs in 2–5% [1, 2]. With increasing numbers of multiple stenoses that are dilated, this complication has become an even greater problem. In most cases, the underlying mechanism is a dissection, resulting in luminal obstruction by an intimal flap [3–5].

Management is difficult, especially in those cases where occlusion occurs hours after angioplasty, when there is no longer an immediate surgical standby available, resulting in a considerable infarction rate due to the time needed until reperfusion is achieved. In addition, acute bypass surgery has a higher mortality than elective operation.

This report describes the experience with a reinterventional approach in this complication of PTCA.

Methods

Strategies in case of acute coronary occlusion after PTCA (Fig. 1)

Patients can be treated conservatively if the occluded vessel is small or if only a side branch of the dilated vessel is occluded. A second option is the acute vein graft operation, provided by the surgical standby. However, as pointed out, this approach still is associated with a high infarction and mortality rate because of the time needed until flow to the occluded vessel is restituted.

An approach possibly resulting in earlier restitution of flow and thus, prevention of infarction, is immediate redilatation. If successful, patients can be managed conservatively. Partial success of redilatation, e.g., antegrade flow but severe residual stenoses, can be followed by semielective CABG-operation.

After unsuccessful redilatation, again there is the option of conservative treatment if surgery is not indicated for other reasons. Secondly, an autoperfusion-catheter can be introduced to provide flow distal to the occlusion. This is followed by immediate CABG-operation. The catheter used in this study had 36 side holes in its distal 10 cm, allowing blood from the aorta to enter the catheter and to perfuse the artery distal to the occlusion, providing more than eight holes on either side of an occlusion, down to an aortic pressure of 50 mmHg.

Another new possible management is the implantation of an intracoronary stent [3]. If the stent keeps the vessel patent, patients can either undergo elective bypass-operation, also using the internal mammary artery, or remain on a conservative treatment. The stent used in this report is a new balloon-expandable, balloon-mounted, tantalum stent with an inflated diameter between 2.5 and 4.0 mm, and the possibility to select diameter in 0.5 mm increments.

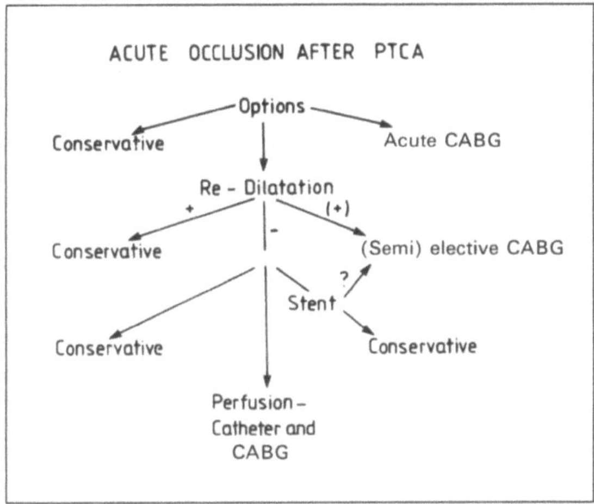

Fig. 1. Therapeutic options in acute coronary occlusions after PTCA.

Patients

In 1500 PTCAs performed between May 1987 and May 1989, we observed 49 (3.3%) acute occlusions, defined as occlusion within 24 h after primarily successful PTCA. Of these 49 patients, 13 underwent immediate CABG-operation, a decision based on immediate availability of an operating team and room, and on presence of multivessel disease in nine patients. Two of them died, one had irreversible left heart failure, one had intracerebral haemorrhage. Ten of them developed a myocardial infarction, six of which were transmural. In the remaining 32 patients, a reintervention was assessed.

Results

In one patient the occluded left anterior descending coronary artery (LAD) could not be reopened; he underwent surgery after a 40 min delay. In 31 patients the occlusion could be crossed by a guidewire and redilated. In ten of them, no permanent patency could be achieved. Three out of these underwent CABG-operation with a deflated balloon in the artery; four of them were operated after introducing an autoperfusion-catheter into the

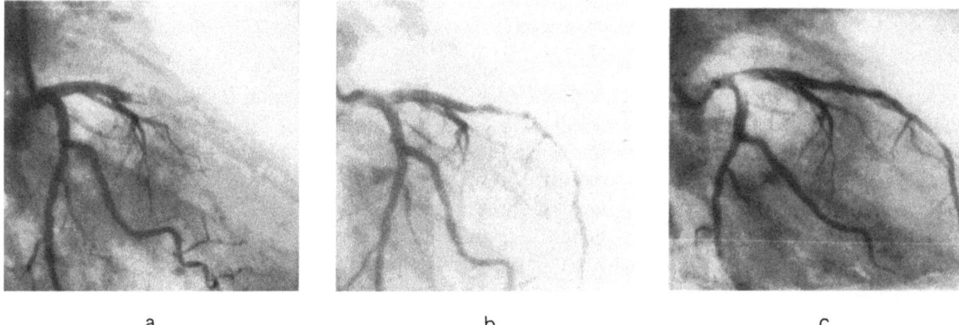

a   b   c

Fig. 2a–c. Coronary angiograms of a case with an occluded LAD 2 h after PTCA (2a) and severe dissection after redilatation (2b) managed by stenting (2c).

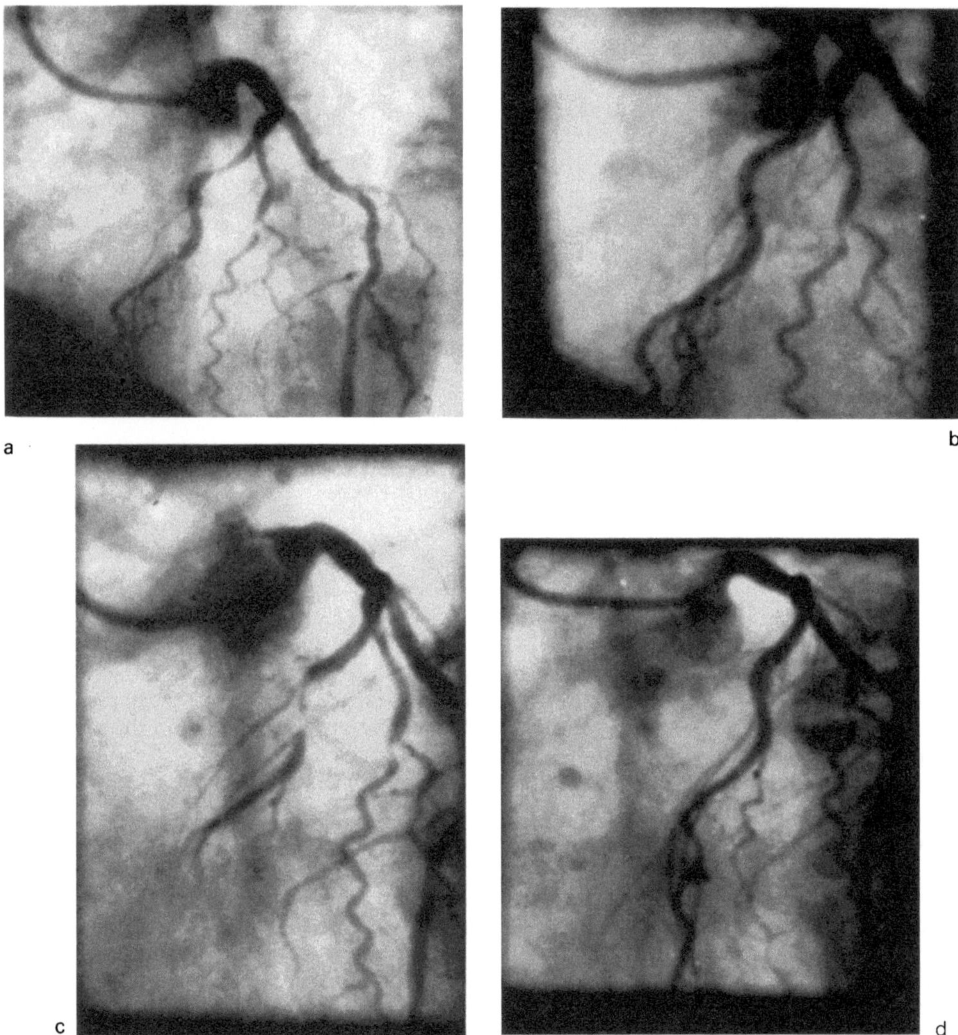

Fig. 3a–d. Shown is a stenosed LAD (3a), primarily dilated with a good result (3b), but occluded 2 h later (3c). In this case, redilatation was successful.

vessel. Two patients with and two without a perfusion catheter (all four with a late occlusion, hours after PTCA) developed a Q-wave myocardial infarction.

In the remaining three patients, for whom no permanent patency could be achieved, a stent was implanted at the dilatation site. All three arteries remained patent. The patients were offered to be operated electively, but all three refused. In Fig. 2, the occluded left anterior descending coronary artery of a patient 2 h after PTCA is shown. This patient had a stent implanted at the occlusion site for heavy dissection, where redilatation alone did not result in permanent patency (Fig. 2b). As can be seen, the stent kept the vessel open (Fig. 2c).

In 20 patients, redilatation was successful. Figure 3 shows the angiograms of a patient with three-vessel disease, who presented with unstable angina. His right coronary and left circumflex coronary artery could be dilated successfully. But while PTCA of his LAD initially was successful as well (Fig. 3a, b) about 2 h after this result was achieved, the patient complained about angina again and the vessel was found to be occluded (Fig. 3c). This case could be managed satisfactorily by redilatation (Fig. 3d).

Up to now, eight patients had repeat angiography within 3 to 9 months because of angina unrelated to the redilated artery. In all eight patients, there was no evidence for restenosis in the redilatated vessel.

In one patient reintervention was only partially successful. The patient had two high-grade LAD stenoses. A first angioplasty had an unsatisfactory result, where only the first stenosis could be crossed and dilated. Twelve hours later acute occlusion of the dilated vessel occurred. On reintervention, the occlusion, as well as the distal stenosis, could be crossed by a "probe". But whereas the proximal lesion could be successfully re-dilated, resulting in immediate antegrade flow, pain relief, and disappearance of ECG-changes, we were unable to dilate the distal stenosis because of a defective balloon that could not be inflated. At this point we decided to abandon the procedure and the patient underwent a semi-elective sequential mammary graft operation to the diagonal branch and the LAD on the following day.

Discussion

Acute coronary occlusion after PTCA constitutes one of the major problems of this technique today. In case of an artery that supplies a large area of the myocardium, in general, emergency bypass grafting is assessed. However, in our patients this strategy is associated with a high rate of myocardial infarctions, confirming other reports in the literature [1].

Given our results, we feel that an reinterventional approach is justified after acute coronary occlusion following PTCA and that it has superior results compared to primary emergency surgery. This holds true especially when newer devices such as the stent are used [3] that enable the interventional cardiologist to handle conservatively even those patients for whom the conventional approach of multiple redilatation fails.

The risk of delaying a surgical revascularization by failure to recross and open the occlusion in our patients is rather low. In only one case surgery was delayed, while the other 31 patients undoubtedly had earlier restitution of bloodflow.

References

1. Simpfendorfer C, Belardi J, Bellamy G, Galan K, Franco I, Hollman J (1987) Frequency, management and follow-up of patients with acute coronary occlusion after percutaneous transluminal angioplasty. Am J Cardiol 59: 267
2. Mabin TA, Holmes DR, Smith HC, Vliestra RE, Bove AA, Reeder GS, Chesbro JH, Bresnahan JF, Orzulack TA (1985) Intracoronary thrombus: Role in coronary occlusion complicating percutaneous transluminal coronary angioplasty. J Am Coll Cardiol 5: 198
3. Sigwart U, Urban P, Golf S, Kaufman U, Imbert C, Fischer A, Kappenberger L (1988) Emergency stenting after coronary balloon angioplasty. Circulation 78: 1121
4. Cowley M, Dorros G, Kelsey S, Van Roden K, Detre K (1984) Acute coronary events associated with percutaneous transluminal coronary angioplasty. Am J Cardiol 53: 12C
5. Block C (1984) Mechanism of transluminal angioplasty. Am J Cardiol 53: 69C

Author's address:
Dr A. Buchwald
Abteilung für Kardiologie
Universitätsklinik
Robert-Koch-Straße 40
3400 Göttingen, FRG

Intracoronary Stents

F. W. Bär, J. van Oppen, H. de Swart, V. van Ommen, P. Leenders, M. Havenith and
E. van der Veen

Dept. of Cardiology and Pathology, Academic Hospital Maastricht, University of
Limburg, The Netherlands

Introduction

Symptomatic coronary artery disease can be treated with medication, coronary artery
bypass grafting (CABG), or percutaneous transluminal coronary angioplasty (PTCA).
However, each of these approaches does have its limitations. At present, several other
developments for the treatment of coronary artery disease are under investigation such as
laser therapy, artherectomy, and stenting of the coronary arteries. The clinical experience
of coronary stenting is limited and does not exceed 600 implants. In this chapter the value
and limitations of the implantation of intracoronary stents will be discussed. Further,
experiences in test animals with a recently developed stent will be presented.

Indications for stent implantation

Stent implantation has been proposed for the treatment of acute occlusive dissections
following a PTCA procedure. Such relatively rare complications (2–5%) will usually result
in myocardial infarction unless adequate therapy is instituted [1, 2, 9, 11, 23]. In case of
single-vessel disease, further intervention is debatable when the dissected artery supplies
only a limited area of myocardial tissue. However, if the ischemic area is more extensive
or multiple-vessel disease is present, the common therapy of choice of this complication
is CABG. To bridge over the delay between the occurrence of the dissection and bypass
grafting, the intermediate treatment is the introduction of a perfusion catheter or frequent
inflations of the balloon catheter at the site of the dissection to restore flow and to prevent
myocardial damage. Another approach to deal with a severe dissection is the implantation
of a stent. This has been shown to be very effective, because the stent compresses the
intimal flap against the vessel wall [20, 21]. Such a back-up device can improve the safety
of PTCA procedures.

Restenosis after PTCA is another problem that is far more frequent. Due to hyperplasia
of the intimal wall, restenosis appears in approximately one-third of the native vessels and
in half of bypass grafts [1, 2, 5, 8, 9]. Earlier reports suggested that stenting might prevent
restenosis.

At the present time, long-term results are rather disappointing and the restenosis [14,
19, 20] rate seems not to be decreased after stent implantation. Therefore, application of
the presently available stents probably should be restricted to acute occlusive dissections
in patients having an elective PTCA. During the first week after the stent implantation,
occlusion due to thrombus formation is the major complication [13, 14, 17–20, 22] for
which aggressive regiments of anticoagulation therapy are given, not uncommonly resulting in bleeding complications. In acute coronary syndromes thrombosis does play an
important role [11]. In such cases stent implantation most likely will result in a significantly
higher occlusion rate.

Table 1. Review of metal stents.

Material	Type of stent	Investigator	(ref)
Nitinol	Thermal shape-memory	Dotter	[6]
Nitinol	Thermal shape-memory	Cragg	[4]
Nitinol	Thermal shape-memory	Sugita	[24]
Stainless steel	Balloon expandable	Palmaz-Schatz	[12]
Stainless steel	Balloon expandable	Roubin	[16]
Stainless steel	Self-expanding (zigzag)	Duprat	[7]
Stainless steel	Self-expanding (multifilament)	Sigwart	[20]
Stainless steel	Self-expanding (double helixspiral)	Maass	[10]
Stainless steel	Self-expanding (parallel wire)	Bär	

Type of stents

Intravascular stents can be divided in three types: memory metal, self-expanding, and balloon deformed stents (Table 1). Materials other than metal have been used, such as Dacron and Gore-tex [15]. Implantation of these nonporous plastic stents resulted in a very high occlusion rate due to thrombus formation. Dotter [6] was the first to implant a coilspring of Nitinol, which is an alloy with thermal shape-memory. The memory metal stents are extremely difficult to handle due to warming during the implantation procedure, as also reported by others [4, 24]. At the present time stents applied in humans are usually composed of stainless steel.

The presently available stents do have such limitations as implantation failure, displacement of the stent, perforation of the vessel wall, poor visibility during implantation, migration of the stent, and spasm of the coronary artery. The stent should be tested for mechanical properties, fatigue of the material, biocompatibility, thrombogenicity, and hemodynamics. Hyperplasia of the intimal wall, which is a frequent finding, probably is the most important problem to consider.

The ideal stent should be macroporous, elastic, radiopaque, easily implantable even in tortuous vessels and absorbable. Further, it should prevent thrombus formation and hyperplasia. To achieve this very difficult and probably impossible task, in vitro and in vivo research has to be performed.

The parallel wire stent and its delivery system

Recently, the parallel wire self-expanding stent (Medtronic Inc. Mineapolis USA) was developed. This stainless steel stent consists of 10 or 12 rods of 0.20 or 0.25 mm (Fig. 1). The ends of the rods are welded by laser light in a zigzag pattern resulting in a cylinder shape. Length of the stent varies between 8 and 12 mm, corresponding to a diameter of 3.0 and 4.5 mm, respectively. For the implantation of the stent a newly developed delivery system is used. This system consists of an inner and outer catheter. The stent is compressed and then loaded at the distal tip of a 4.2 or 4.9 French outer catheter. Then the system is moved to the implantation area over an 0.014-inch guide wire, the inner catheter is advanced until it abuts against the stent, after which the outer catheter is withdrawn. The stent is freed and allowed to expand (Fig. 1).

Experimental model

The stents were implanted in normal coronary arteries of young and healthy pigs. We used this preparation because of its better similarity to humans in regard to coronary artery size

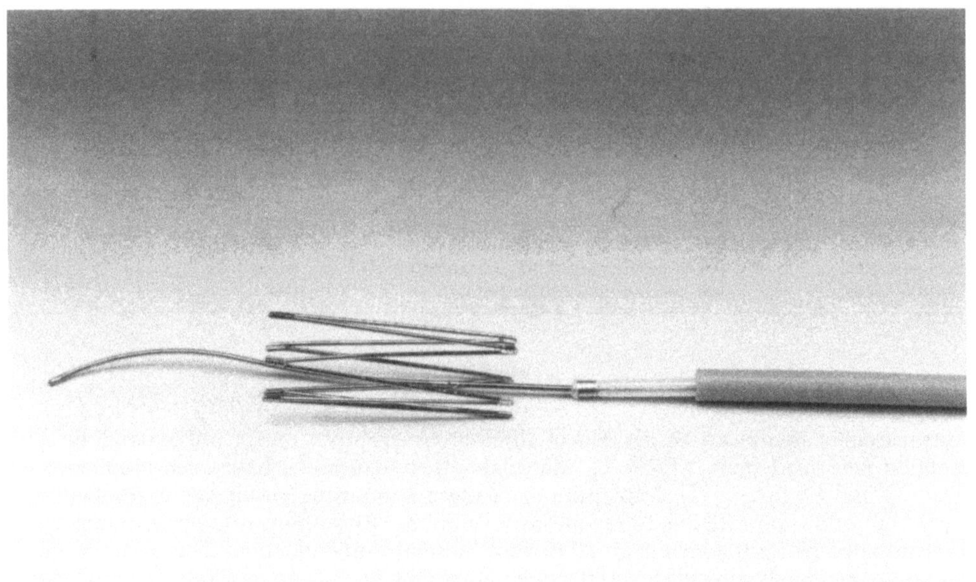

Fig. 1. The stent and the inner and outer catheter of the delivery system.

and clotting mechanism. We tested the stents in coronary arteries to investigate the behavior of the stents in the most difficult environment: a moving contractile object.

The animals had pretreatment with sublingual nifedipine and antibiotics. During the procedure, heparine and intracoronary nitroglycerine was injected. After the implantation, no further therapy was given in order to test thrombogenicity of the stent. Fluoroscopy was performed the next day to study possible migration of the stent. To investigate potential early stenosis, cardiac catheterization was repeated at 1 and 3 weeks, after which the animal was sacrificed and the coronary arteries were dissected for macroscopic and microscopic investigation.

Results

Thirty-three stents were implanted in the normal coronary arteries of 17 pigs. Right coronary artery: 15 stents; left anterior descending artery: 10 stents; circumflex artery: eight stents. Diameter of the stent was chosen to be approximately 0.5 mm larger than the diameter of the vessel. Implantation of the stent at a predetermined site was accurate, rapid, and easy in 31 of 33 stents. Two stents were incorrectly positioned in small side branches. Both mistakes can be explained by the low resolution of the x-ray device and the lack of a motor-powered injector. Immediately after implantation, due to spasm, poor flow was seen in one of the two stented side branches. Three other pigs also had coronary spasm immediately after the procedure, as was observed at the electrocardiogram and the control angiogram.

Intracoronary nitroglycerine was effective in two of these three animals; the third pig subsequently died. Another pig died several hours later for reasons unknown. Autopsy of both animals revealed open arteries and a non-occlusive thrombus in one stented artery.

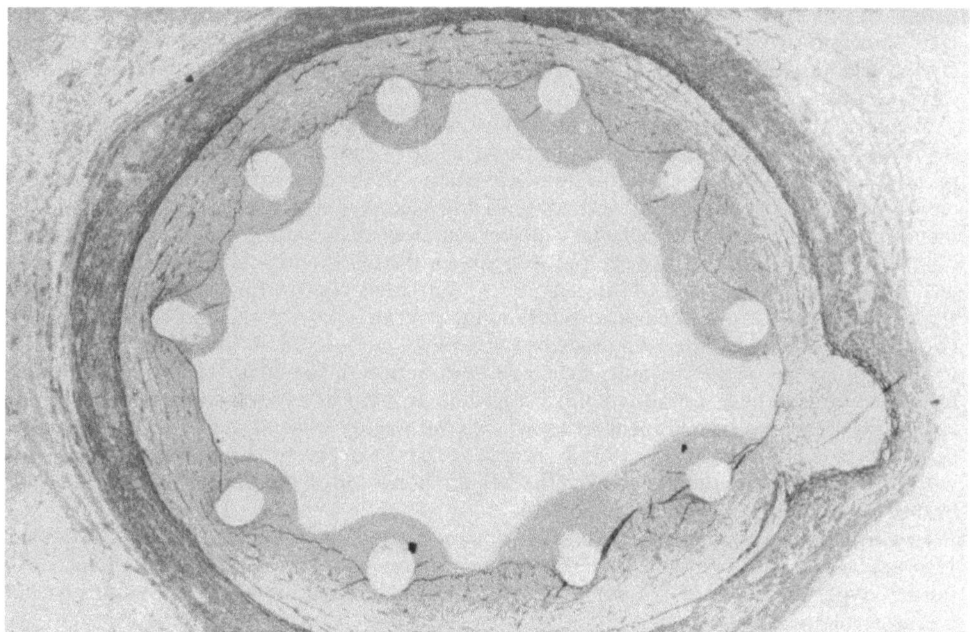

Fig. 2. Elastin van Gieson stained cross-sectioned stented coronary artery. All rods of the stent are imbedded in a neointimal layer.

During the first week, three other animals died – one pig due to a bleeding due to a puncture of the jugular vien, the other due to ventricular fibrillation during intubation. Microscopy revealed that the stented coronary arteries of these two swine were widely open. The third pig had an occluded stented side branch and probably died due to the right ventricular infarction (confirmed at autopsy).

During follow-up at one and three weeks, all 25 stented vessels were open in the remaining 13 animals. However, spontaneous migration of two stents was observed in spite of adequate sizing. This finding might be related to the vasomotor tone of the coronary artery. The other 23 stents had expanded well; all stents were exactly in their original locations. In addition to the third angiogram the animals were sacrificed.

Autopsy confirmed results of angiography at one and three weeks. Macroscopically, no thrombus was seen in the stented areas. The stents were well attached against the vessel wall and side branches were open. Microscopically, the rods were fully covered by a neointimal layer. No important hyperplasia was present at this time (Fig. 2); mean percentage of stenosis due to the rods and hyperplasia was 20% (range 0–30%).

Discussion

Several types of stents are under investigation (Table 1). The Medivent stent introduced by Sigwart [20] and the Palmaz-Schatz stent [12, 13, 17–19] are in clinical evaluation. Both types of stents meet the problems of (sub)acute thrombosis and intimal hyperplasia. The parallel wire stent is a more recent development; it is, however, not tested in humans. This stent partially resembles the Gianturco stent [7, 16, 25, 26]. In our hand, the parallel wire stent is usually easy to implant, and others [3] have had the same experience. Short-term results of this stent were reasonably good. At three weeks, small non-occlusive thrombi were found in two pigs, coronary flow was not impaired. This is of particular interest as testing was done in animals in whom no anticoagulant therapy was administered after implantation.

Weighed against other presently available stents, the parallel wire stent has its limitations. Implantation failure and malplacement have been observed. Visibility of the compressed stent is good, but it is poor after expansion. An optimal catheterization laboratory environment will probably prevent some of the mistakes which occurred in our experiments. Perforation of the coronary artery leading to severe complications was not observed. Spasm was the most common problem during the experiments. However, it is well known that, compared to humans, even pretreated pigs do have a high incidence of spasm. An interesting finding was spontaneous migration out of the coronary arteries of two stents, which have not been described in animals or humans so far. Whether vasomotor tone or spasm of the coronary artery or contraction of the heart itself are responsible for this complication is unknown. Only a limited amount of hyperplasia was observed. It can be expected that intimal proliferation will continue up to 8–10 weeks. Then, stabilization or even some regression of the hyperplasia can be expected. Long-term experiments with this stent are now in progress. Whether the behavior of the parallel wire is different in diseased arteries of humans is unclear.

In contrast to some other stents, this device is rigid, which might be less favorable. However, one can speculate that flexibility may come with the disadvantage of excessive intimal hyperplasia [19]. The stent is short, but multiple implantations can be done within a reasonable time.

Conclusions

It has been demonstrated that implantation of intracoronary stents is feasible and is a welcome addition in the treatment of severe dissections. The parallel wire stent might represent a valuable adjunct to these stents. Nevertheless, the presently used "first generation" stents do have a rather high complication rate. The most frequent (sub)acute clotting problems have decreased after initiation of rigid anticoagulation protocols. Long-term results indicate that restenosis cannot be prevented by presently available stents. Stents might even enhance hyperplasia of the intimal wall. Therefore, restenosis rates probably are more or less identical in patients with and without stents. New designs are mandatory for treating hyperplasia of the intimal wall.

References

1. ACC/AHA Task Force on assessment of diagnostic and therapeutic cardiovascular procedures (subcommittee on Percutaneous Transluminal Coronary Angioplasty) (1988): Guidelines for percutaneous transluminal coronary angioplasty. Circulation 78: 486
2. Bertrand ME, Marco J, Cherrier F, Schmidt R, et al. (1986) French percutaneous transluminal coronary angioplasty (PTCA) registry: Four years experience. J Am Coll Cardiol 7-21A
3. Bonan R, Bhat K, Ki Leung T, et al. (1989) The self-expanding wire metallic stent. J Am Coll Cardiol 13: 106A
4. Cragg A, Lund G, Rysavy J, et al. (1983) Non-surgical placement of arterial endo-prosthesis: A new technique using Nitinol wire. Radiology 147: 261
5. Dorros G, Johnson W, Tector AJ, et al. (1984) Percutaneous transluminal coronary angioplasty in patients with prior coronary artery bypass grafting. J Thorac Cardiovasc Surg 87: 17
6. Dotter CT (1969) Transluminally-placed coilspring endo-arterial tube grafts: long-term patency in canine popliteal artery. Invest Radiol 4: 329
7. Duprat G, Wright KC, Charnsangavej Ch, Wallace S, Gianturco C (1987) Self-expanding metallic stents for small vessels: an experimental evaluation. Radiology 162: 469

8. Faxon DP, Sanborn TA, Weber VJ, et al. (1984) Restenosis following transluminal angioplasty in experimental atherosclerosis. Arteriosclerosis 4; 189

9. Grüntzig AR, King SB, Schlumpf M, Siegenthaler W (1987) Long-term follow-up after percutaneous transluminal coronary angioplasty. N Engl J Med 316: 1127

10. Maass D, Zollikofer ChL, Largiadèr F, Semming A (1984) Radiological follow-up of transluminally inserted vascular endoprosteses: An experimental study using expanding spirals. Radiology 152: 659

11. Mabin TA, Holmes DR Jr, Smith HC, et al. (1985) Intracoronary thrombus: Role in coronary occlusion complicating percutaneous transluminal coronary angioplasty. J Am Coll Cardiol 5: 198

12. Palmaz JC, Windeler SA, Garcia F, et al. (1986) Atherosclerotic rabbit aortas: expandable intraluminal grafting. Radiology 160: 723

13. Palmaz JC, Garcia O, Kopp DT, et al. (1987) Balloon Expandable intra-arterial stents: effect of anticoagulation on thrombus formation. Circulation suppl 76: IV 45

14. Puel J, Joffre F, Rousseau H, et al. (1987) Endo-prostheses coronariennes auto-expansives dans la prevention des restenoses apres angioplastie transluminale. Arch Mal Coeur 164: 709

15. Ring EJ, Schwarz W, McLean GK, Freiman (1982) A simple, indwelling, biliary endoprosthesis made from commonly available catheter material. AJR 139: 615

16. Roubin GS, Robinson KA, King III SB, et al. (1987) Early and late results of intracoronary arterial stenting after coronary angioplasty in dogs. Circulation 76: 891

17. Schatz R, Palmaz JC, Tio FO, et al. (1987) Balloon-expandable intracoronary stents in the adult dog. Circulation 76: 450

18. Schatz RA, Palmaz JC (1989) Balloon Expandable Intravascular Stents (BEIS) in human coronary arteries: A follow-up report 61st Scientific Sessions. J Am Coll Cardiol 13 (II): 106A

19. Schatz A (1989) A view of vascular stents. Circulation 79: 445

20. Sigwart U, Puel J, Mirkovitch V, Joffre F, Kappenberger L (1987) Intravascular stents to prevent occlusion and restenosis after transluminal angioplasty. New Eng J of Med 316: 701

21. Sigwart U, Urban P, Svein G, et al. (1988) Emergency stenting for acute occlusion after coronary balloon angioplasty. Circulation 78: No 5, 1121

22. Sigwart U, Golf S, Kaufmann U, Kappenberger L (1988) Analysis of complications associated with coronary stenting. J Am Coll Cardiol II: 66A

23. Simpfendorfer C, Belardi J, Bellamy G, et al. (1987) Frequency, management and follow-up of patients with acute coronary occlusion after percutaneous transluminal angioplasty. Am J Cardiol 59: 267

24. Sugita YU, Shimomitsu T (1986) Non-surgical implantation of a vascular ring prosthesis using thermal shape memory Ti/Ni Alloy (nitinol wire). Trans Am Soc Artif Intern Organs 32: 30

25. Uchida BT, Putnam JS, Rösch J (1988) Modifications of Gianturco expandable wire stents. AJR 150: 1185

26. Wright KC, Wallace S, Charnsangavej CH, Carrasco CH, Gianturco C (1985) Percutaneous endovascular stents: An experimental evaluation. Radiology 156: 69

Author's address:
Frits W. Bär, Cardiologist
Department of Cardiology
Academic Hospital of Maastricht
P.O. Box 1918
6201 BX Maastricht
The Netherlands

Surgery after Complications of PTCA: An Overview on Strategy, Techniques, and Results

J. Ennker, H. Warnecke, G. Reinicke and R. Hetzer

German Heart Institute, Berlin, FRG

Introduction

Guidelines of the American Heart Association [8] and of the German Society for Cardiac and Circulatory Research (Deutsche Gesellschaft für Herz- und Kreislaufforschung) [7] both exclude patients from PTCA in whom myocardial infarction of life-threatening severity would follow an occlusion of the stenosis to be dilated. However, a certain rate of severe complications after PTCA seems to be inevitable, due to the unpredictable clinical course of an individual patient once myocardial ischemia has been produced [3]. The amount of myocardium at risk does not predict the severity of complications to be expected, because other factors such as arrhythmias, distribution of thrombembolic material, and extending dissection may suddenly convert a situation of stable ischemia into a catastrophic hemodynamic deterioration. It appears that even the most thoughtful indication for PTCA cannot completely rule out the need for emergency coronary surgery. A review of the surgical experience will outline our present surgical view of the problem.

Ischemic time interval

Once ischemia has occurred, it is not possible to define a safe time-limit for successful revascularization without myocardial infarction for an individual patient. In patients with stable circulation and good left ventricular function, with sufficient collateral blood supply to the area of myocardium at risk, reperfusion within 2 h will often result in an outcome without infarction [21, 23]. If, however, left ventricular function is compromised, filling pressures are elevated, catecholamine medication is required, and arrhythmias further reduce cardiac output and myocardial perfusion ischemia tolerance of the myocardium may be minimal. The risk of entering a vicious cycle of ventricular distension and dysfunction, cardiogenic shock, and life-threatening arrhythmias is high, and surgical reperfusion must be accomplished within a very short time [5, 16]. An average below 45 min between onset of ischemia and start of extracorporeal circulation could be reached in our institution in patients with PTCA complications (Table 1). Operative results in this group were superior to results after longer ischemic intervals. In our experience, one patient (4.76%) out of 21 patients with time intervals below 45 min died. Above that, the operative risk rose to 22%. If cardiopulmonary resuscitation was necessary before extracorporal circulation, the risk was 38%. Satter reports an infarction rate of 70% and a mortality of 12.6% in patients with persistent transmural ischemia, whereas intermittent ischemia resulted in an infarction rate and mortality below 6%. Most authors report an influence of ischemic time interval on outcome with regard to infarction rate [21] and survival [6, 13, 20, 23]. Conclusions can also be drawn from former studies on revascularization of acute myocardial infarction, where the success of surgical reperfusion of infarcted myocardium depends on the time interval elapsed [6, 18]. A further time-related risk factor is the observation that patients requiring cardiopulmonary resuscitation often do

Table 1. Results of emergency revascularization in the German Heart Center, Berlin.

From April 1986 to May 1989; total of 48 patients	N	+	%
Time interval < 45 min up to start of surgery	21	1	4.76
Time interval > 45 min up to start of surgery	27	6	22.22
Cardiopulmonary resuscitation before bypass	13	5	38.46
Previously operated patients	2	2	100
Total	48	7	14.50

not do so initially after the PTCA complication, but do so after a time interval that could have been used to prepare surgery and to install cardiopulmonary bypass.

Summarizing the above experience, management after complicated, failed PTCA has to be highly time conscious. Surgical standby is valid only if patient transport is well organized and no undue delays occur with the induction of surgery. There is no safe time interval before surgery, and mortality and infarction rate are correlated to the time loss before surgical reperfusion. Time intervals quoted in the guidelines of respective associations [7] or in the literature are arbitrary and do not justify any delay.

The upper time-limit of successful revascularization in a stable patient is under debate. Probably, periods of ischemia far beyond a 2 h limit can still be survived with viable myocardium left intact. Periods of 6 h or more of persistent ischemia probably are too long for successful revascularization [6].

Surgery versus percutaneous recanalization

Surgical revascularization after coronary occlusion by PTCA carries inherent problems, which are not present if a trial of re-opening the vessel by catheter procedures is successful. Surgery requires cardioplegic arrest of the heart, which can be induced without loss of myocardial function only if myocardial energy stores are preserved and ATP levels are near normal. Induction of cardioplegic arrest in the presence of depleted myocardial energy stores, as may be the case after resuscitation or high-dose catecholamine medication, will not protect the myocardium, but may result in additional functional damage. Cases not weanable from cardiopulmonary bypass mainly fall in this category. Therefore, it appears advisable to fully exploit catheter techniques for percutaneous recanalization and for maintaining flow distal to an occlusion before surgery [11, 15, 22]. Catheter recanalization, even if successful, is only temporary, but it does improve the outlook for myocardial recovery after surgery and should be applied whenever technically possible. Experience shows that even minimal perfusion of a large coronary artery with hand-held syringes can prevent perioperative myocardial infarction. Generally, surgeons should request that flow be maintained to distal coronary arteries during transportation and induction of anaesthesia. With up-to-date equipment, surgery in the presence of nonperfused occluded large coronary arteries should no longer be necessary.

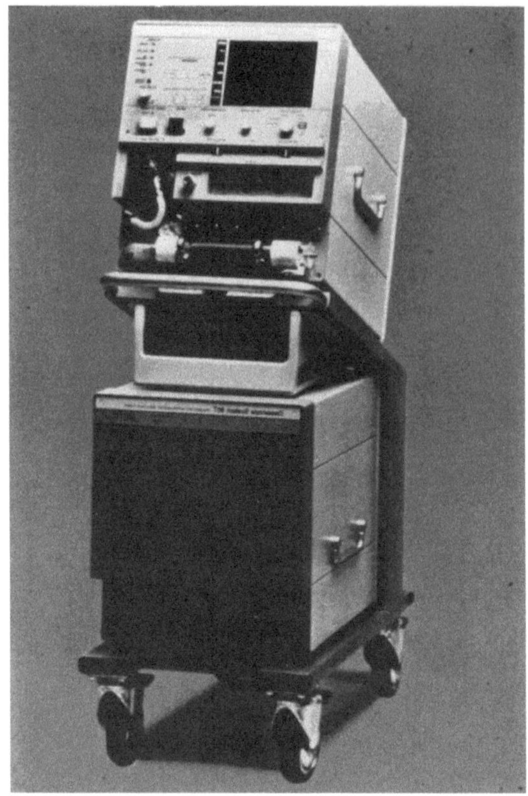

Fig. 1. Transportable intraaortic balloon
pump.

Intraaortic balloon pump support

The use of intraaortic counterpulsation is more often advocated than it is used in the
setting of hemodynamic instability. IABP support certainly can help in stabilizing
hemodynamics by afterload reduction and improved diastolic coronary perfusion. The
primary goal should be immediate surgical reperfusion, however, it is uncertain whether
the myocardium distal to a PTCA-induced occlusion benefits from balloon pumping. The
results of balloon pumping in primary acute myocardial infarction illustrate that balloon
pumping in itself does little to salvage myocardium and its purpose can only be to bridge
the circulation until surgery [1, 14, 16, 17]. Installation of the balloon requires time, even
with the percutaneous catheter systems available today, or may be impossible in patient
with iliac artery occlusive disease. Furthermore, patient transport by emergency vehicles
between separate units or buildings is difficult. The small transportable balloon pumps
available may help in this situation (Fig. 1). In our own experience, we are well aware of
the potential benefits of balloon support, but we only advocate it when there is minimal
time loss with insertion and the patient cannot immediately be put on cardiopulmonary
bypass. Often connection to the heart-lung machine is performed in a time span not much
longer than required for placement of the balloon. If, however, preparation of the
operating room or other measures can be expected to consume some time, the lag time is
well spent on insertion of a balloon.

116

Surgical considerations

In emergency bypass grafting the risk for myocardial damage is localized in the ischemic regions, but there is also the risk of global myocardial depression initiated by low output, high filling pressures, reduced coronary perfusion, and ventricular distension. These factors support each other and may lead to a vicious cycle that causes near total energy depletion of the myocardium [16].

Thus, surgical management is not only directed towards reperfusion of myocardium at risk in the shortest possible time, but also has to achieve decompression of the cardiac chambers as soon as possible. Revascularization can be handled like routine coronary surgery in most cases, with the exception of use of the internal mammary artery as discussed below, and it must be kept in mind that temporary hemodynamic stability does not justify any delay, because infarction rate and the need for resuscitation are time-dependent events. Immediate decompression of cardiac chambers requires special considerations, otherwise the situation of a reperfused coronary system with global heart failure, induced by prolonged ventricular distension before cardioplegic arrest, may not be uncommon. For this reason we do not favor connection of the patient to extracorporal circulation with percutaneous cannulae in the catherization laboratory. By these cannulae, pump flows up to 4 liters/min can be reached, however, distension of the heart is not relieved and the metabolic state of the myocardium will worsen during the time necessary for the procedure. In patients who reach the operating room in stable hemodynamic condition, it should be possible to open the chest and install extracorporal circulation with direct drainage of heart chambers quickly, thus creating much better conditions for functional myocardial recovery after cardioplegic arrest. However, if the patient is already under resuscitation, instantaneous extracorporal circulation via femoral cannulation is advisable in order to maintain continuous adequate cerebral and cardiac perfusion. In the next step, median sternotomy is performed and decompression of the heart via the right atrium and a left ventricular vent catheter is obtained.

Patients after previous cardiac surgery present a special problem. These patients can be quickly supported with extracorporal circulation via femoral cannulation, but sometimes require considerable operative time for access to the heart. During this interval, decompression of the left ventricle cannot be achieved and risk of global myocardial damage is high. Both patients in our experience could not be weaned from extracorporal circulation.

Mechanical circulatory support

Present extracorporal technology allows the emergency initiation of full-flow extracorporal circulation in patients in cardiogenic shock or under cardiopulmonary resuscitation. With expertise, this can be achieved within a few minutes. The indication for the various techniques of access for connection of the heart-lung machine, however, depends on the clinical status and the therapeutic perspective of the patient.

Access by puncture of femoral vessels

This technique allows cannulation of extracorporal circulation via percutaneous cannulae in the catheter laboratory. It should be considered, however, as a rescue procedure only, because pump flow is restricted and does not always allow full support of the circulation. There is no decompression of the failing left ventricle, which makes consecutive bypass surgery hazardous.

Femoral access for extracorporal circulation

Under resuscitation or in reoperations, it is preferable to use the femoral artery and vein for cannulation. Full circulatory support is possible, however, decompression of the heart cannot be achieved until thoracotomy is performed. Under cardiopulmonary resuscitation, the femoral approach allows continued cardiac massage until extracorporal circulation is established.

Access by median sternotomy

This is the preferred approach in all situations excluding resuscitation or previous cardiac surgery.

Ventricular assist devices

The use of ventricular assist devices (Fig. 2) requires extracorporal circulation for implantation. At present, the indication is restricted to patients after emergency revascularization if severe ventricular dysfunction makes the patient pump-dependent or if the patient has the prospect of receiving a heart transplant after recovery of noncardiac organ function [9]. Support of a failing heart in a patient who has permanent contraindications for transplantation is not a promising approach. In rare situations after satisfactory revascularization, support may be used to permit functional recovery of the heart with subsequent weaning from pump support.

Perioperative infarction rate

For planning a therapeutic schedule for a patient amenable to PTCA, it must be kept in mind that most authors judge the results of emergency coronary surgery to be inferior to an elective coronary artery bypass graft procedure in a comparable patient. The perioperative infarction rate is high [2, 3, 17, 18, 21] and must be expected to be between 20% and 50%. Three-vessel disease and diffuse coronary disease carry the highest risk of perioperative myocardial infarction [9, 21] and of unsatisfactory late outcome [4]. This risk is prohibitively high in left main stenosis and most surgeons do not agree on stand-by in this situation. Only occasionally are infarction rates reported that are comparable to those after elective coronary surgery [10].

Long-term results

The major technical determinant of long-term success after coronary surgery is the use of the internal mammary artery. Patients in whom the left internal mammary artery has been used have a better long-term patency rate and a longer survival than comparable patients with saphenous vein grafts alone [12]. The policy with regard to use of the mammary artery is under debate. Most surgeons prefer not to use the mammary artery, as this would further increase the bleeding risk which is already high due to the administration of platelet inhibitors and thrombolytic substances in most patients. In addition, preparation of the internal mammary artery requires more time than harvesting a bypass graft vein. However, Ferguson [10] reported on a large series of emergency patients with evolving

118

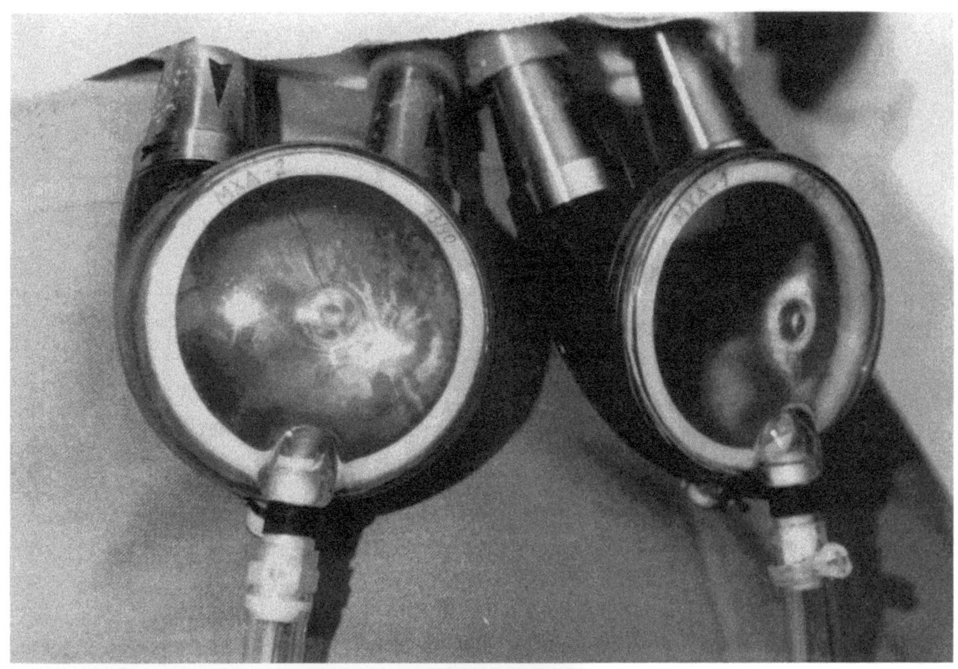

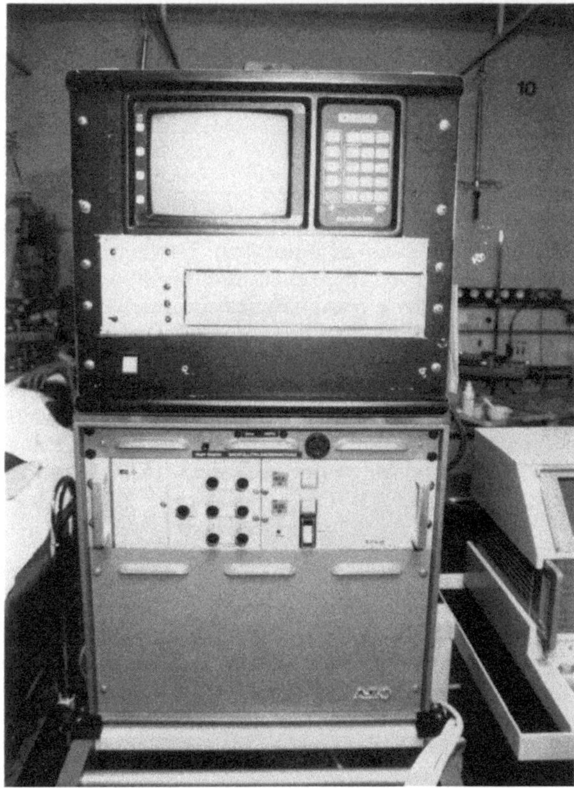

Fig. 2. Ventricular assist device, the "Berlin Heart".

119

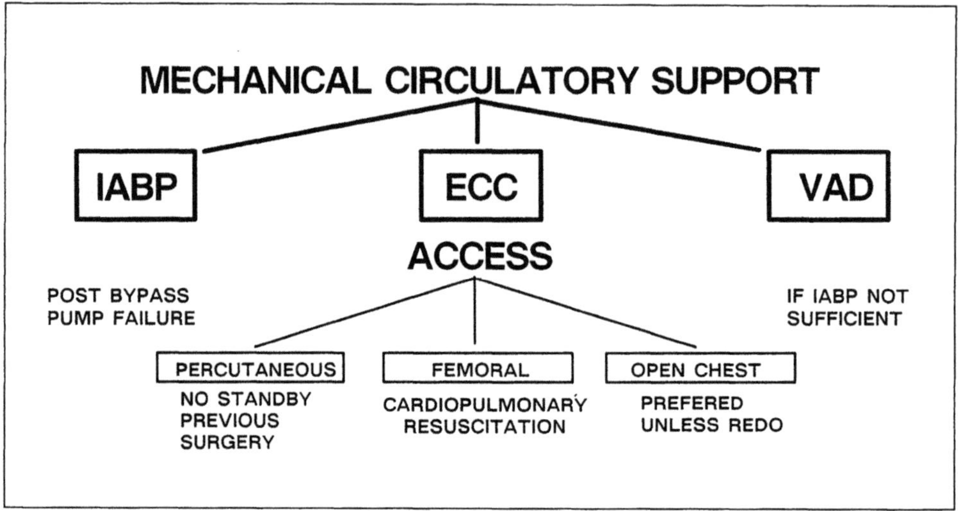

Fig. 3. Mechanical circulatory support. (Abbrevations: IAPB = intraaortic balloon pump; EEC = extracorporal circulation; VAD = ventricular assist device)

myocardial infarction where the internal mammary artery has been used with good success, although the rate of postoperative bleeding was substantial, as was to be expected under these conditions. We advocate use of the mammary artery only if extracorporal circulation has reestablished a normal ECG as an indicator that the extra time required does not prolong critical ischemia, and we would then perform the dissection of the mammary artery on extracorporal circulation to prevent hemodynamic instability.

Patient transport and induction of anaesthesia

Within the same institution, patient transport with arterial blood-pressure monitoring and, eventually, an intraaortic balloon pump should not be a problem. This is not the case if an ambulance or helicopter has to be used. However, arterial continuous blood pressure monitoring appears mandatory and can be done by a portable pressure monitor. Transportation with a running balloon pump requires more time and cannot be recommended if blood pressure can be maintained by medication. Even with advanced models of a transportable balloon pump, we would fear a loss of time and potential complications if transport to another hospital becomes necessary. We normally request that the cardiologist familiar with the patient's coronary anatomy accompanies the patient during transport for support of the emergency medical staff and for communicating with the stand-by surgical team.

Conclusion

Acute ischemia as a result of failed PTCA leads to an unfavorable situation for successful surgical revascularization. Emergency bypass grafting often has to be done under time constraints in unstable patients, or under cardiopulmonary resuscitation. The metabolic state of the myocardium (not just in the area of impending infarction) is compromised by high filling pressures and maximum energy turnover that stresses the viable myocardium.

120

Table 2. Comparison of results after emergency PTCA.

	PTCAs	Emergency operation	AMI	Deaths
Bredlau	3502	92 (2.7%)	47 (51%)	2 (2.0%)
Brahos	323	68 (21.0%)	–	3 (4.4%)
Parsonnet	958	67 (7.0%)	19 (28.3%)	8 (11.9%)
Pelletier	265	35 (13.2%)	10 (28.6%)	0
Satter	1633	82 (5.0%)	44 (53%)	9 (10.9%)

This impairs myocardial protection by cardioplegic arrest which is necessary for the surgical procedure. Consequently, metabolic and functional recovery of the myocardium after cardioplegic arrest can be compromised. Thus, the surgeon's primary goal is to minimize aortic clamp time. Revascularization as an emergency procedure cannot be compared to an elective procedure. With regard to operative risk, rate of perioperative myocardial infarction and completeness of revascularization results are inferior (Table 2). This requires careful indications for the PTCA procedure, primarily in order to prevent the need for surgical intervention.

Parsonnet et al. justifiably have stated: "Because emergency operation after failed angioplasty carries with it significant postoperative morbidity and mortality, this procedure cannot be considered equivalent to elective coronary bypass grafting" [19].

References

1. Bardet J, Rigaud M, Kahn JC, Huret JF, Gandjbakhch, Bourarias JHP. (1977) Treatment of post-myocardial infarction angina by intraaortic balloon pumping and emergency revascularization. J Thorac Cardiovasc Surg; 74:299
2. Brahos GJ, Baker NH, Ewy HG, Moore PJ, Frankhauser DM. (1985) Aortocoronary bypass following unsuccessful PTCA: Experience in 100 consecutive patients. Ann Thorac Surg; 40:7–10
3. Bredlau CE, Roubin GS, Leimgruber PP, Douglas JS, King SB, Gruentzig AR. (1985) In-hospital morbidity and mortality in patients undergoing elective coronary angioplasty. Circulation; 72:1044–52
4. Connor AR, Vliestra RE, Schaff HV, Ilstrup DM, Orszulak TA. (1988) Early and late results of coronary bypass after failed angioplasty. J Thorac Cardiovasc Surg; 96:191–97
5. Cox JL, McLaughlin VW, Flowers NC. (1968) The ischemic zone surrounding acute myocardial infarction. Its morphology as detected by dehydrogenase staining. Am Heart H; 76:650
6. De Wood MA, Spores J; Berg R, Kendall RW, Grundwald RP, Selinger SL, Hensley GR, Sutherland KI, Shields JP. (1983) Acute myocardial infarction: A decade of experience with surgical reperfusion in 701 patients. Circulation; 68 (Suppl II):II 8–16
7. Empfehlungen für die Durchführung der perkutanen transluminalen Koronarangioplastie (PTCA). Z Kardiol 1987; 76:382–85
8. Executive Committee of the NHLBI PTCA Registry. (1982) Guidelines for the performance of PTCA. Circulation; 66:693–94
9. Farrar DJ, Hill JD, Gray LA, Pennington DG, McBride LR, Pierce WS, Pae WE, Glenville B, Ross D, Galbraith TA, Zumbro GL. (1988) Heterotopic prosthetic ventricles as a bridge to cardiac transplantation: A multicenter study in 29 patients. N Engl J Med; 318:333–40
10. Ferguson TB, Muhlbaier LH, Salai DL, Wechsler AW. (1988) Coronary bypass grafting after failed elective and failed emergent percutaneous angioplasty. J Thorac Cardiovasc Surg; 95:761–72
11. Ferguson TB, Hinoharo T, Simpson J, Stack RS, Wechsler AS. (1986) Catheter reperfusion to allow optimal coronary bypass grafting following failed transluminal coronary angioplasty. Ann Thorac Surg; 42:399
12. Kirklin JW, Naftel DC, Blackstone EH, Pohost GM. (1989) Summary of consensus concerning death and ischemic events after coronary artery bypass grafting. Circulation; 79 (Suppl I):I 82–91
13. Krebber HJ, Mathey DG, Kuck KJ. (1982) Management of evolving myocardial infarction by intracoronary thrombolysis and subsequent aorto-coronary bypass. J Thorac Cardiovasc Surg; 83:186–93

14. Leinbach RC, Gold HK, Dinsmore RE, Mundth ED, Buckley MJ, Austen WG, Sanders CA. (1973) The role of angiography in cardiogenic shock. Circulation; 47–48 (Suppl III):95
15. Marquis JF, Schwartz L, Aldridge H, Majid P, Henderson M, Matushinsky E. (1984) Acute coronary artery occlusion during percutaneous transluminal coronary angioplasty treated by redilatation of the occluded segment. J Am Coll Cardiol; 4:1268–71
16. Mundth E. (1983) In: Sabiston DC, Spencer F (eds). Gibbon's Surgery of the chest; 1490–1515
17. Murphy DA, Craver JM, Jones EL, Curling PE, Guyton RA, King SB, Gruentzig AR, Hatcher CR. (1984) Surgical management of acute myocardial ischemia following percutaneous transluminal coronary angioplasty. Role of the intra-aortic balloon pump. J Thorac Cardiovasc Surg; 87:332–39
18. Norell AS, Lyons J, Layton C, Balcon R. (1986) Outcome of early surgery after coronary angioplasty. Br Heart J; 55:223–26
19. Parsonnet V, Fisch D, Gielchinsky I, Hochberg M, Hussain SM, Karanam R, Rothfeld L, Klapp L. (1988) Emergency operation after failed angioplasty. J Thorac Cardiovasc Surg; 96:198–203
20. Pelletier LC, Pardini A, Renkin J, David RP, Herbert Y, Bourassa MG. (1985) Myocardial revascularization after failure of percutaneous transluminal coronary angioplasty. J Thorac Cardiovasc Surg; 90:265–71
21. Satter P, Krause E, Skupin M. (1987) Mortality trends in cases of elective and emergency aortocoronary bypass after percutaneous transluminal coronary angioplasty. Thorac Cardiovasc Surgeon; 35:2–5
22. Schofer J, Krebber HJ, Bleifeld V, Mathey DG. (1982) Acute coronary occlusion during percutaneous transluminal angioplasty: reopening by intracoronary streptokinase before emergency coronary artery surgery to prevent myocardial infarction. Circulation; 66:1325–31
23. Wilson JM, Dunn EJ, Wright CB, Bailey WB, Callard GM, Melvin DB, Mitts DL, Will RJ, Flege JB. (1986) The cost of simultaneous surgical standby for percutaneous transluminal coronary angioplasty. J Thorac Cardiovasc Surg; 91:362–70

Author's address:
Dr. J. Ennker
Deutsches Herzzentrum Berlin
Herz-Thorax-u. Gefäßchirurgie
Augustenburger Platz 1
1000 Berlin 65, FRG

Restenosis after Angioplasty

Restenosis following Coronary Angioplasty

K. J. Beatt, P. W. Serruys

Academic Department of Cardiovascular Medicine, Charing Cross and Westminster
*Hospital, London, U.K. and Thoraxcenter, Erasmus University, Rotterdam, The
Netherlands

Introduction

With the high initial success rates that are regularly reported for coronary angioplasty it
has become increasingly difficult to demonstrate methods or techniques that are able to
provide more beneficial acute results than can be achieved by conventional angioplasty.
On the other hand, the incidence of late restenosis has remained much the same over the
10 years that angioplasty has been part of clinical practice [1] and there is still no proven
intervention which modifies the restenosis process. The problem of restenosis has therefore
assumed increasing relevance in determining the clinical value of coronary angioplasty,
and accordingly, studies that address the problem of restenosis have needed to become
more exacting. Although there have numerous articles addressing the problem of restenosis in the clinical setting, with many defining certain factors associated with restenosis
and possible interventions to reduce the incidence of restenosis, there is surprisingly little
consensus. Most of the discrepancies can be attributed to three factors: 1) the selection of
patients, 2) the method of analyis, 3) the definition of restenosis employed. The purpose
of this review is to show that these three factors influence the outcome and conclusions of
restenosis studies.

The long-term clinical outcome will remain important in assessment. However, the most
objective means of assessing restenosis following angioplasty is by carefully controlled
coronary angiography at the time of the procedure and at a defined follow-up time. In the
past, visual estimation of the angiographic films was used but a consensus is now beginning to emerge that recognises the limitation of this approach. The use of a quantitative
angiographic measuring system for assessing both the immediate and the long-term results
of therapeutic interventions such as angioplasty appears mandatory.

Metholological considerations

There are currently many studies on restenosis reported in the literature which are
dintinguished by their lack of consistency in their methodological approach, their definition of restenosis and the reported factors influencing restenosis.

These studies are demanding in terms of time and financial resources and are also
demanding on the patient as, at least for the time being, there is a need to repeat
angiography even if the patient is asymptomatic. This is because of the reported incidence
of silent restenosis which may be as high as 33% if a sensitive-enough index is used [2].
It is important, particularly with studies that look at the impact of a new intervention on
restenosis, that their design is capable of showing the effect of the intervention if indeed
one exists. Many of the studies published so far have failed to be sufficiently exacting to
form a basis for their conclusions. In order to improve the situation there are in principle
three areas which need to be addressed:

This work was supported by grants from: The Netherlands Heart Foundation, The Hague, The Netherlands; The British Heart Foundation, London U.K., and the Wellcome Trust, London, U.K.

1) Population; if the results are intended to apply to the angioplasty population, then the study population must reflect this. This means a high angiographic follow-up rate with invididual patients time-to-restudy being predetermined at the time of angioplasty, and not influenced by the recurrence of symptoms or the anatomy of the lesion post-angioplasty. This will avoid a selection bias of symptomatic patients, or patients with orderline post-angioplasty results.

It can be estimated that if a 30% reduction in the restenosis rate is to be realised at the 0.05 significance level with a power of 0.80, then in a double-blind randomised study 400 patients will be needed in each of the placebo and active treatment groups. For a 50% reduction in restenosis then 150 patients will be needed in each group to obtain the same statistical certainty. Many studies that conclude by showing no benefit of a particular intervention do not include a sufficient number of patients to show a benefit if indeed one exists.

2) A well-validated system of analysis with known accuracy and variability should be employed. The use of a visual, percentage-diameter-stenosis measurement with its inherent variability precludes meaningful results while edge-tracing by hand or other techniques which can produce values that are not physiologically possible are also unacceptable.

3) The measured parameters must be chosen so as to reflect the restenosis process and distinguish between the results of angioplasty and this process. The conventional assessment of percentage-diameter-stenosis is not sufficiently discriminating to do this, since when there is a concomitant decrease in the reference or normal diameter of the vessel, a smaller lumen may have a larger measured percentage-diameter-stenosis.

The behaviour of the dilate following angioplasty

The use of quantitative angiography has provided valuable insights into the problems of assessing restenosis, and it has exposed many of the false premises surrounding the topic. Figure 1 shows the mean angiographic data from 490 lesions assessed at different follow-up intervals between 1 and 5 months following angioplasty. Early following angioplasty there is little change in the mean values of the minimal luminal diameter, the reference diameter or the percentage-diameter-stenosis, with individual lesions showing both significant improvement and deterioration. The individual changes in minimal luminal diameter of these lesions are represented in the frequency histogram shown in Fig. 2. The progressive shift of the distribution of the minimal luminal diameter with time to follow-up is evident and shows that it is not just a limited number of lesions that "restenose", but rather, almost all lesions deteriorate to some extent by 120 days post-angioplasty. This is suggested by the "shift" of the curve and it is the inherent variability of measurement which gives a distribution showing some lesions improving and most deteriorating. This is a concept that is not well understood in the context of restenosis. The degree of change is normally distributed about their respective mean ($-0.42\,\text{mm}$ at 120 days) and the number of lesions that "restenose" will depend on the criterion chosen. The presence of intimal dissection or mural thrombus at the time of the procedure, as well as the occurrence of delayed recoil, will all influence the assessment of late "restenosis". Just how important each of these factors is, is uncertain as there is little information on the outcome of the dilated lesion over the first 48 h, although the information that is available suggests a significant number of lesions deteriorate in this early period [2]. At 3 months the deterioration in the lesions becomes significant for the group, with the restenosis rate peaking at 25–37% depending on the criterion used, as shown in Fig. 3. A significant deterioration is also seen in the reference diameter which tends to minimise the change in the measured percentage diameter stenosis [3] (Fig. 4). Further progression after 6 months is unusual, with lesion improvement or deterioration occurring in a small number of instances – a pattern more characteristic of coronary artery disease in general [4–6].

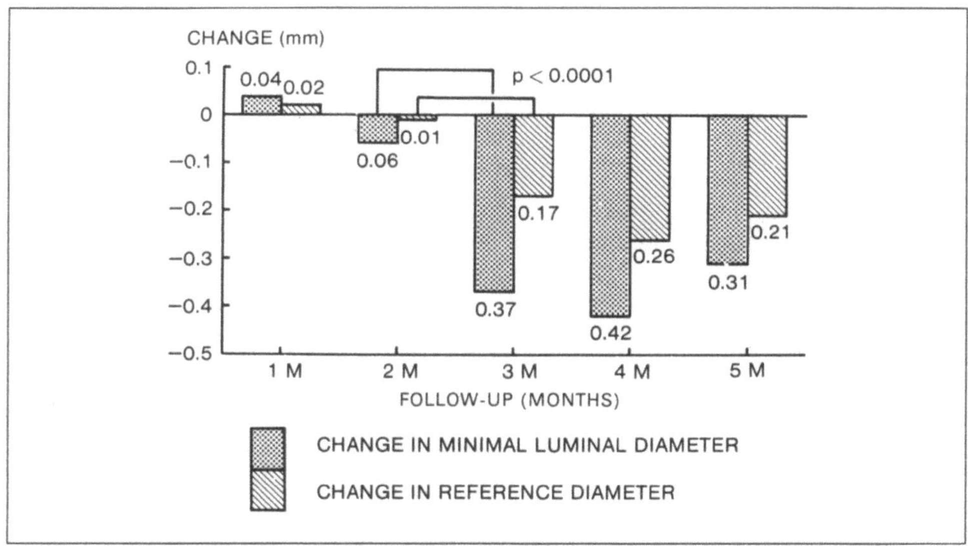

Fig. 1. Mean change in reference diameter and minimal luminal diameter for the five follow-up groups. At 90, 120 and 150 days both these changes are significant ($p \geqslant 0.0001$).

It seems likely that the restenosis process begins early and is progressive over the first 3–4 months. The limitations of even the most accurate measurement systems mean that these early changes are not detected early, and it is not until substantial progression takes place at 3 months that the process is fully recognised. This early change has been shown in animals where there is evidence of smooth muscle proliferation as early as 7 to 14 days following dilation [7]. This same process has been identified in at least seven post-mortem hearts [8–10] that were examined over a period of 17–150 days post-angioplasty.

Incidence of restenosis

While accurate assessment suggests that the trend to restenosis applies to most of dilated lesions, deciding which of these lesions should be defined as restenosis is less clear. The restenosis definition of choice has been the subject of much debate and there is currently no satisfactory definition that takes into account both the functional and angiographic outcome of the patient after PTCA. The confusion and controversy that surround the subject of restenosis are essentially due to four factors. The first is that many angiographic definitions try to combine the angiographic outcome with a clinical outcome. The known discrepancy between these two parameters means that this objective will not be realised, particularly in multivessel disease. Secondly, a single "stenosis" measurement should not be confused with a measurement of "restenosis" that should represent the change in stenosis severity. Thirdly, criteria which are defined by a cut-off value at follow-up or which are biased by the improvement in lesion diameter obtained at angioplasty, will preselect those lesions with a less satisfactory result post-angioplasty. Fourthly, definitions based on percentage diameter stenosis measurements may fail to identify lesions undergoing significant deterioiration. These criteria are chosen to reflect the change in mimimal luminal diameter in relation to the so-called normal diameter of the vessel in the immediate vicinity of the obstruction. It also assumes that this "normal diameter" (or the reference diameter) of the vessel, proximal or distal to the obstruction does not change, either as a

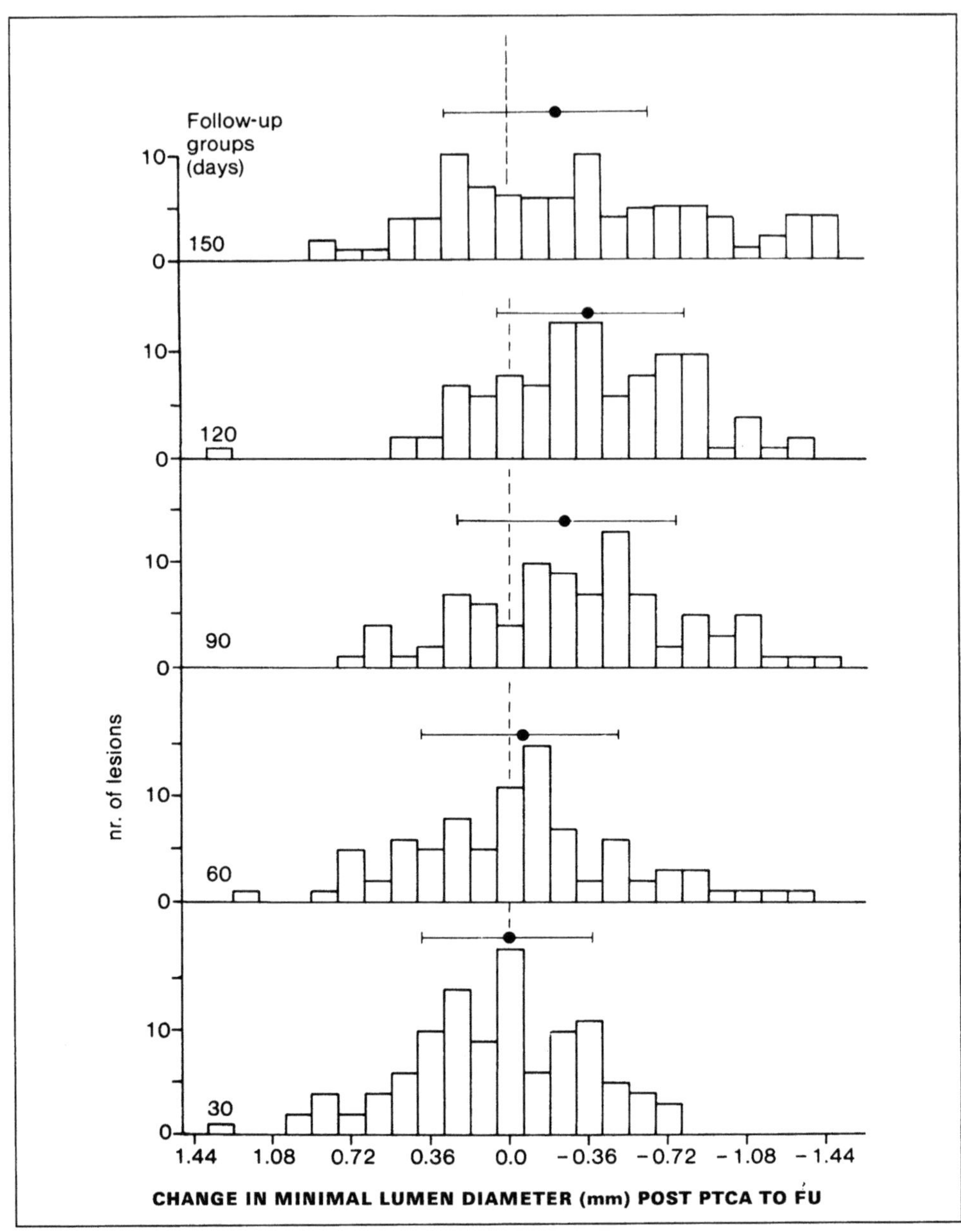

Fig. 2. Histograms for the five follow-up groups showing the distribution in the change of minimal luminal diameter with time. The vertical interrupted line represents no change, and the mean for each group and one standard is also represented.

result of angioplasty or during the immediate follow-up period, when restenosis of the dilated lesion is a well-recognised phenomenon. Quantitative angiographic studies have shown this premise to be false. This seriously questions the use of percentage-diameter-stenosis as the only index of restenosis [2,3].

128

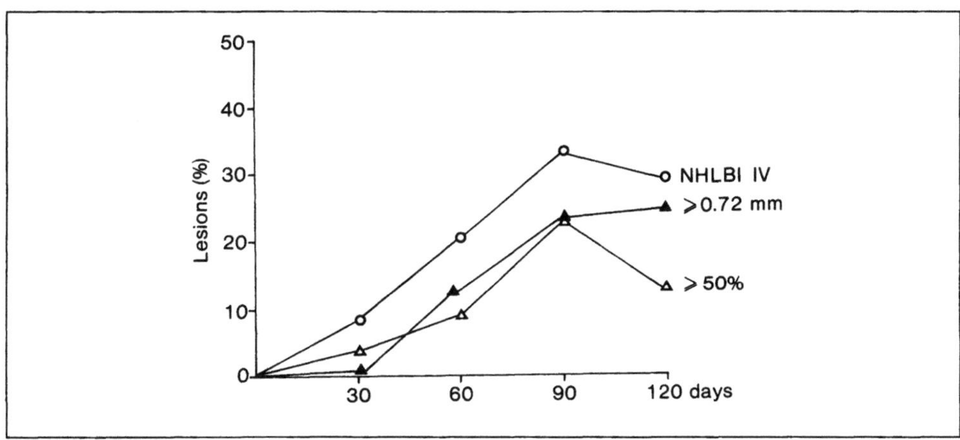

Fig. 3. The incidence of restenosis according to three different criteria in the first 120 days following angioplasty derived from a patient population of 490 successfully dilated lesions. (M = months, see Fig. 3 for other abbreviations).

Bearing in mind the above mentioned points, what is the rationale for the restenosis criteria in current use? Most are entirely arbitrary, some are based on doubtful logic and some, although of some relevance for visual estimation of percent-diameter-stenosis, are unrealistic when applied to the more accurate values obtained from quantitative angiography.

The definitions of restenosis used in major restenosis studies are:

1) Loss of at least 50% of the initial gain achieved at angioplasty [11];

2) A return to within 10% of the pre-angioplasty diameter stenosis [12];

3) An immediate post-angioplasty diameter stenosis of less than 50% that increases to 50% or greater at follow-up [12,13];

4) As for 3), but for a diameter stenosis of 70% or greater at follow-up [14];

5) Deterioration of 0.72 mm in minimal luminal diameter or greater from post-angioplasty to follow-up [15];

6) Deterioration of 0.5 mm in minimal luminal diameter or greater from post-angioplasty to follow-up [2].

If we examine the commonly used definition of $\geqslant 50\%$ DS at follow-up, this is historically based on the physiological concept of coronary flow reserve and is taken because it represents the approximate value in animals with normal coronary arteries at which a blunting of the hyperemic response occurs [16]. Although this value may be of some relevance in determining a significant stenosis in human atherosclerotic vessels it tells us nothing about the way the lesion has behaved since the angioplasty procedure.

As a result of quantitative angiographic studies a new concept for defining restenosis criteria based on the change in minimal lumen diameter has been introduced [5] (Fig. 4). The change in this value from post-angioplasty to follow-up can be expected to give a good quantitative measurement of the degree of restenosis. The restenosis criterion or the cut-off point dividing the restenosis group from the non-restenosis group is then derived by determining the variability of measurement (1 SD of the differnece in means) of the same lesion taken from separate catheter sessions. Twice the variability (95% confidence intervals) defines with reasonable certainty those lesions that have undergone significant deterioration from those that have not. Reiber et al. have found this value to be 0.72 mm based on angiograms taken 90 days apart [17], whereas Nobuyoshi et al., using a different

129

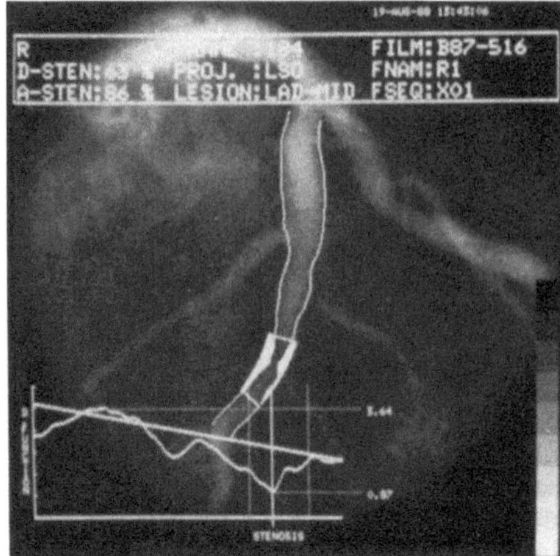

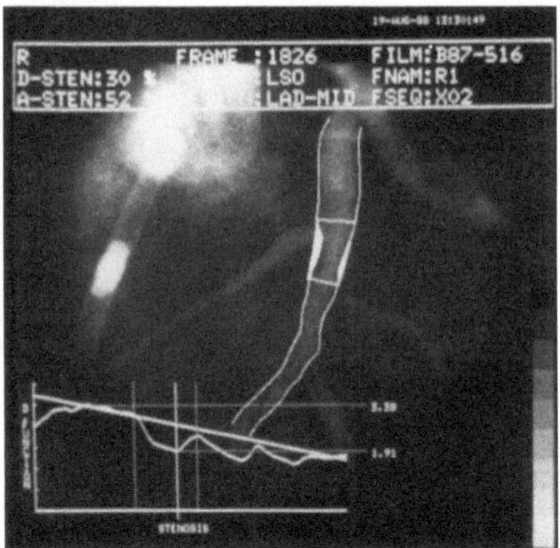

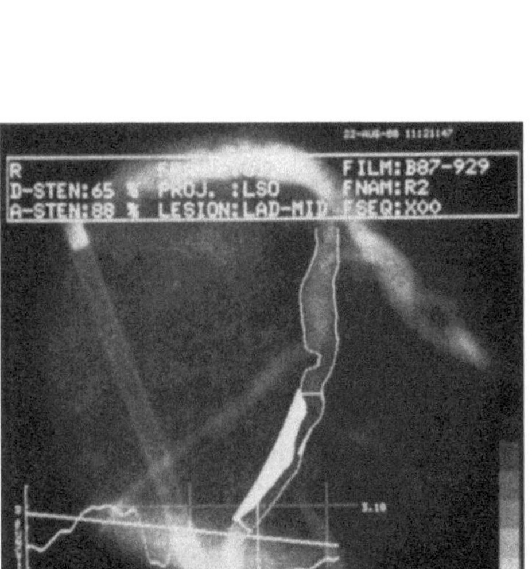

Fig. 4. Shown are a series of single-frame angiograms of a left anterior descending coronary artery pre-dilation, post dilation and at follow-up. Quantitative coronary analysis was performed using CAAS. The arterial boundaries detected by the systems are shown on the angiogram, and below the diameter function curve, derived from these contours.

The example is chosen to illustrate the difficulty and importance in choosing appropriate reference diameter. Although the lesion is relative discrete, the tapering of the vessel (due to frequent side branches before, within, and immediately after the lesion) make the pre-angioplasty choice of reference diameter difficult. At follow-up the fact that the dilated but non-stenotic coronary artery is involved in the restenosis process, and that the length of the lesion has increased magnifies the problem. By using the interpolated reference diameter derived from the interpolated diameter function line (the line sloping downwards from left to right on the diameter-function tracing) these problems, although not entirely resolved, are minimised and are at least standardised. This gives a more appropriate value for the percentage-diameter-stenosis, but does not give an appropriate indication of the degre of stenosis, which in this case is extensive and severe.

measurment system, have taken 0.5 mm based on angiograms taken 7–10 days apart [2]. It is important to realise that the variability will be considerably greater for angiograms taken from repeat catheterisation sessions, as opposed to repeat angiograms from the same session [17], something that has not been appreicated by all investigators using this methodology.

Criteria based on the absolute change in minimal luminal diameter are, nevertheless, limited as they make no attempt to relate the extent of the restenosis process to the size of the vessel. What may be a significant increase in plaque area in a 1.5 mm diameter vessel, may be of no hemodynamic consequence in a larger vessel of 3.5 mm. Studies need to be undertaken to assess the variability of measurement in different diameter vessels, and a "sliding scale" criteria must be set that adjusts for vessel size.

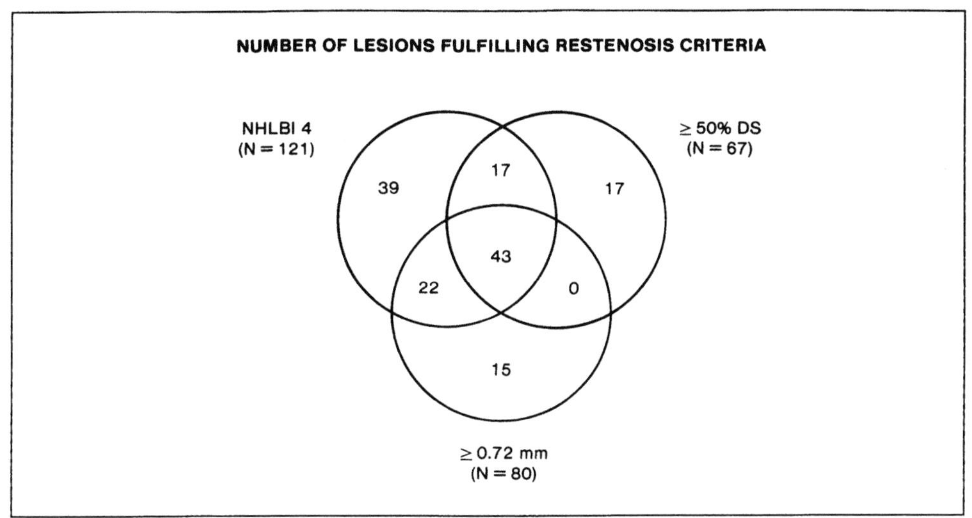

Fig. 5. Illustrated are the number of lesions fulfilling three different restenosis criteria, taken from a population of 490 lesions followed up within 6 months. The total number of lesions that fulfil each criterionare shown under that criterion and none others are enclosed by only one circle.

Lesions included by any two criteria are enclosed by two circles, and lesions that fulfil all three criteria (n = 43) are enclosed by all three circles. It can be seen that lesions that are designated as restenosis are highly dependent on the criterion for restenosis employed. (NHLB14 = criterion 4 of the National Heart, Lung and Blood Institute: loss of greater than 50% of the gain at angioplasty; ≥ 50% DS = ≥ 50% diameter stenosis at follow-up; ≥ 0.72 mm = ≥ 0.72 mm change from post-angioplasty to follow-up).

Figure 5 shows the number of lesions fulfilling three different criteria of restenosis, although 43 of the lesions included by at least one criterion are included by all three; 32% of those included in one of the criterion ("a loss of greater than half the gain") are not included in either of the other two. Despite this discrepancy the incidence of restenosis is not too dissimilar, ranging from 21% to 34% as shown in Fig. 3. What should be clear is that a similar incidence of restenosis with different criteria may be defining different populations. This point has particular relevance when determining the risk factors for restenosis; if restenosis cannot be reliably determined, then it is unlikely that the associated risk factors will be identified.

The most sensitive index of restenosis in common use is that of a loss of ≥ 50% of the gain with reported incidences ranging from 16% to 52% [11,12,15,18]. However, ≥ 50% diameter stenosis at follow-up will tend to give a lower incidence of restenosis because lesions that deteriorate significantly but remain within the 0–49% range are not designated as restenosis. Of the two studies with large numbers which document the change in minimal lumen diameter, only one uses this value to derive a restenosis value of 26% at 4 months [15].

The use of quantitative aniography has given valuable insight into the problem of defining an incidence of restenosis. It has been demonstrated that the restenosis process takes place to some extent in most of the lesions dilated and, furthermore, it takes place in not only the stenotic portion, but also in the dilated but non-stenotic segments [3]. This observation in itself demands the use of a measurement system that will define the change in the minimal luminal diameter independent of the change in the "reference diameter".

Risk factors for restenosis

There are no studies using quantitative coronary angiography that report on the risk factors in large number of patients. There are some factors relating to the restenosis process that have been identified and confirmed in more than one study. These include a proximal left anterior descending coronary artery stenosis, a totally occluded vessel pre-angioplasty, the presence of collaterals supplying the distal part of the dilated coronary artery and associated insulin-dependent diabetes. Factors that relate to the success of the angioplasty such as residual stenosis of greater than 30% or 40%, should not, with current knowledge, be considered as risk factors for "restenosis". For most of the other described risk factors it seems that there are as many studies that do not identify a particular factor as studies that do identify them. No procedural-related factor which would allow the operator to modify the way in which the angioplasty procedure is performed has yet been identified, and no pharmacological intervention has been able to show a reduced rate of restenosis. Quantitative angiography offers the possibilty of objective measurement of lesion morphology such as length of lesion and eccentricity, and when this more objective information becomes available then, perphaps, it will be possible to identify lesion-related factors associated with restenosis.

To date, clinical restenosis studies have provided us with little information on how to effectively modify the restenosis. What they have done is to better define the problem of restenosis in the clinical setting, and to make us more aware of our current limitations. It seems likely that with better measurement systems, particularly those that can be online in the catheterisation laboratory, it will be easier to perform these studies, and with more reliable data in smaller number of patients, the effects of various interventions to prevent restenosis will be more accurately and more efficiently assessed. There are currently a wide variety of revascularization devices, procedures and pharmacological interventions under investigation, and of crucial importance in their evaluation will be the restenosis rate associated with each of these strategies. It is already clear that a meaningful comparison between the various strategies and evaluation of their relative merits is not possible due to a lack of standardisation of methodology and lack of objectivity. In the future, we should demand that quantitative analysis be employed in important studies addressing the long-term outcome of new coronary interventions, so that the present confusion is not perpetuated.

References

1. Gruentzig AR, Senning A, Siegenthaler WE (1979) Non operative dilation of coronary artery stenosis: percutaneous transluminal coronary angioplasty. N Engl J Med 301: 61
2. Nobuyoshi M, Kimura OT Nosaka H (1988) Restenosis After Successful Percutaneous Transluminal Coronary Angioplasty: Serial Angiographic Follow-Up of 299 Patients. J Am Coll Cardiol 12: 616–23
3. Beatt KJ, Luijten HE, de Feyter PJ (1983) Change in diameter of coronary artery segments adjacent to stenosis following percutaneous transluminal coronary angioplasty: Failure of percentage diameter stenosis measurement is reflect morphological charges induced by balloon dilation. J Am Coll Cardiol; 12: 315–23
4. Kramer JR, Kitazuma H, Proudfit WL, Matsuda Y, Williams GW, Sones FM. (1983) Progression and regression of coronary atherosclerosis: Relation to risk factors. Am Heart J 105: 134–144
5. Bruschke AVG, Wijers TS, Kolsters W, Landmann J, et al. The anatomic evolution of coronary artery disease demonstrated by coronary arteriography in 256 patients. Circulation 1981; 63: 527–36
6. Kramer JR, Matsuda Y, Mulligan JC, Aronow M, Proudfitt WL. Progression of coronary atherosclerosis. Circulation 1981; 63: 519–25
7. Steel PM, Chesebro JH, Stanson AW, Holmes DR Jr, Dewanjee MK, Badimon L, Fuster V. (1985) Balloon angioplasty. Natural history of the pathophysiological response to injury in a pig model. Cir Res 57: 105–12

8. Essed CE, van den Brand M, Becker AE. (1983) Transluminal coronary angioplasty and early restenosis: Fibrocellular occlusion after wall laceration. Br Heart J 49: 393–6
9. Waller BF, McManus BM, Gorfinkel JH, et al. (1983) Status of the major epicardial coronary arteries 80 to 150 days after percutaneous transluminal coronary angioplasty. Analysis of necropsy patients. Am J Cardiol 51: 81–84
10. Austin GE, Ratiff NB, Hollman J, Tabei S, Phillips DF. (1985) Intimal proliferation of smooth muscle cells as an explanation for recurrent coronary artery stenosis after percutaneous transluminal coronary angioplasty. J Am Coll Cardiol 6: 369–375
11. Thornton MA, Gruentzig AR, Hollman Y, King SB, Douglas JS, et al. Coumadin and aspirin in the prevention of recurrence after transluminal coronary angioplasty: a randomised study. Circulation 1984; 69: 721–727
12. Leimgruber PP, Roubin GS, Hollman J, Cotsonis GA, Meier B, Douglas JS, King III SB, Gruentzig AR. Restenosis after successful coronary angioplasty in patients with single-vessel disease. Circulation 1986; 73: 710–7
13. Holmes DR, Vlietstra RE, Smith HC, Vetrovec GW, Kent KM, Cowley MJ, Faxon DP, Gruentzig AR, Kelsey SF, Detre KM, Raden MJ van, Mock MB. (1984) Restenosis after percutaneous transluminal coronary angioplasty (angioplasty): A report from the PTCA Registry of the National Heart, Lung, and Blood Instistute. Am J Cardiol 53(2): 77C–81C
14. Corocos T, David PR, Val PG, et al. (1985) Failure of Diltiazepam to present restenosis after percutaneoous transluminal coronary angioplasty. Am Heart J 109: 926–931
15. Serruys PW, Luijten HE, Beatt KJ, et al. Incidence of restenosis after successful coronary angioplasty: a time-related phenomenon. Circulation 1988; 77: 361–371
16. Gould KL, Lipscombe K. (1974) Effects of coronary stenoses on coronary flow reserve and resistance. Am J Cardiol 33: 87–94
17. Reiber JHC, Serruys PW, Kooijman CJ, Wijns W, et al. Assessment of short-, medium-, and long-term variations in arterial dimensions from computer-assisted quantitation of coronary cineangiograms. Circular 2985; 71: 280–8
18. Levine S, Ewels CJ, Rosing DR, Kent KM, et al. (1985) Coronary angioplasty: Clinical and angiographic follow-up. Am Cardiol 55(6): 673–676

Author's address:
K.J. Beatt MD
Department of Cardiovascular Medicine
Charing Cross and Westminster Medical School
Horseferry Road
London SW1P 2AP, UK

Factors Correlating with Restenosis after PTCA

H. J. Rupprecht, R. Brennecke, R. Erbel and J. Meyer

Second Medical Clinic, Johannes Gutenberg University, Mainz, FRG

Introduction

Since its introduction in 1977 [7, 8], PTCA has been widely used in patients with coronary artery disease. Restenosis with recurrence of angina remains the major problem, limiting the long-term success after PTCA. Reported restenosis rates vary from 17% to 47% [9–19, 22–26]. In larger series [12, 15, 26] a restenosis rate of about 30% was constantly found, irrespective of the definition of restenosis in use.

But there is still much controversy about the risk factors that predispose to restenosis. So far, only few studies have analyzed a sufficiently large number of patients and risk factors by multivariate analysis. An early report of the National Heart, Lung and Blood Institute (NHLBI-Registry) selected four variables, associated with an increased rate of restenosis [12]. None of these variables was confirmed in a larger series of Emory University [15] where they revealed five other factors independently related to an increased risk of restenosis. Moreover, only limited data are available on procedure-related factors such as inflation time, number of inflations, and inflation pressure. Therefore, we evaluated our data in patients with single-vessel disease and follow-up angiography to determine the risk factors for the development of restenosis.

Patients and methods

Between January 1983 and January 1988, a first PTCA procedure was performed in 768 patients with single-vesel disease. Patients with left main disease, chronic total occlusion, acute myocardial infarction or previous aorto-coronary bypass grafting had been excluded from the study. A stenosis > 50% was present in all patients. During the procedure a surgical team was available in case of need. Informed consent was obtained from all patients. The procedure was performed according to the technique of Grüntzig [7, 8], via the femoral route. The severity of coronary lesions was measured at the maximum percentage diameter narrowing in any standard angulation.

The angioplasty procedure was considered to be successful in 676 patients (88%) with a reduction of at least 20% in luminal diameter narrowing and a post-PTCA stenosis < 50% without the patient having major complications.

In 473 of all successfully dilated patients (70%), repeat coronary angiography was performed as recommended at a mean of 6 months after the initial PTCA procedure. These patients were evaluated in the following with regard to risk factors for restenosis. There was no significant difference between patients with and without follow-up with regard to baseline characteristics. Restenosis was defined as a) loss of > 50% of the initial gain in luminal diameter and b) a luminal diameter narrowing > 50%.

Statistical analysis

All variables evaluated as risk factors are listed in Table 1. Differences in categorical variables were assessed by Chi-square analysis. Continuous variables were categorized

Table 1. Possible risk factors for restenosis.

Clinical variables:	Age, sex, angina-class (CCS), unstable angina, duration of symptoms; history of smoking, diabetes mellitus, hypertension, hypercholesterinemia; previous myocardial infarction.
Angiographic variables	
pre-PTCA:	Severity of stenosis before PTCA, length of stenosis, eccentricity, site of stenosis with regard to the dilated vessel, site of stenosis with regard to proximal, medial or distal location, calculated normal diameter at the site of stenosis.
post-PTCA:	Residual stenosis after PTCA, improvement of stenosis, intimal dissection.
Procedural variables:	Maximal inflation pressure, maximal single inflation time, total inflation time, number of inflations, ratio of balloon diameter/vessel diameter.

CCS = Canadian Cardiovascular Society Classification.

with respect to the subsequent multivariate analysis. In a subgroup of 458 patients in whom a complete set of data was available, multivariate analysis was performed using a stepwise logistic regression model.

A p-value < 0.05 was considered to indicate a relevant difference.

Results

Overall results

Restenosis, as defined above, was found in 138/473 patients (29%) after successful PTCA. The mean diameter stenosis amounted to $26.9 \pm 15.6\%$ in patients without restenosis compared to $78.1 \pm 13.9\%$ in the restenosis group (p = 0.0001).

Risk factors for restenosis

Clinical risk factors: Patients with unstable angina were at higher risk of restenosis (Table 2) than patients with stable angina (38% vs 25%, p = 0.004). A short duration of symptoms (< 1 month) was associated with a significantly higher restenosis rate, compared to patients with a longer history of angina symptoms (44% vs 25%, p = 0.005). A slightly higher rate of restenosis was found for male sex (30% vs 25%), Diabetes mellitus (33% vs 28%), age > 60 years (36% vs 28%) and angina class III and IV compared to class I and II (32% vs 25%) without reaching statistical significance. Other clinical risk factors had no influence on restenosis.

Angiographic variables (pre-PTCA)

A high grade stenosis $> 90\%$ before PTCA was followed by a restenosis rate of 37%, as compared to 19% if the pre-PTCA stenosis measured $< 70\%$ (p = 0.014, Table 2). Accordingly, we found a recurrence rate of 35% in stenoses with a free lumen $< 0.4\,\text{mm}$ as compared to 21% in stenoses with a free lumen $> 0.8\,\text{mm}$ before PTCA (p = 0.033). Distal lesions had a recurrence rate of 27% compared to 32% in proximal lesions (ns). No

Table 2. Univariate analysis of risk factors for restenosis.

Variable	n	Rate of restenosis (%)	p value
Duration of angina			
< 1 month	25/57	44	0.005
≥ 1 month	86/338	25	
Angina			
stable	81/326	25	0.004
unstable	55/145	38	
Initial stenosis (%)			
< 70%	23/119	19	
70–90	84/270	31	0.014
> 90	31/84	37	
Initial stenosis (mm)			
< 0.4	45/130	35	
0.4–0.8	62/197	31	0.033
> 0.8	31/146	21	
Residual stenosis (%)			
< 15	34/166	20	
15–30	36/148	24	0.001
> 30	68/159	43	
Residual stenosis (mm)			
< 2.0	49/111	44	
2.0–2.5	51/187	27	0.001
> 2.5	38/175	22	
Improvement of stenosis (%)			
< 50	63/175	36	
50–70	49/188	26	0.042
> 70	26/110	24	
Improvement of stenosis (mm)			
< 1.5	59/175	34	
1.5–2.0	44/144	31	0.083
> 2.0	35/154	23	
Maximal single inflation time (s)			
< 30	41/166	25	
30–60	69/236	29	0.017
> 60	24/53	45	
Total inflation time (s)			
< 120	25/93	27	
120–240	57/222	26	0.055
> 240	52/140	37	
Maximal inflation pressure (atmospheres)			
< 7	111/346	32	0.028
≥ 7	23/109	21	

other pre-PTCA angiographic variables such as length, eccentricity, or diseased vessel were significantly correlated with restenosis.

Angiographic variables (post-PTCA)

A residual stenosis < 15% immediately following the PTCA procedure was combined with a restenosis rate of only 20%, whereas a residual stenosis > 30% was subject to a 43% recurrence rate (p = 0.001, Table 2). Again the above data correlated with measurements of the absolute stenosis diameter after PTCA. In stenoses with a free lumen < 2 mm after PTCA, the restenosis rate amounted to 44% as compared to 22% if the residual

Table 3. Multivariate stepwise logistic regression analysis of risk factors for restenosis.

Variable	Beta	Std. Error	Beta/ Std. Error	p	Increased risk of restenosis
Stenosis after PTCA	0.56639	0.13448	4.21170	0.0001	Large residual stenosis
Maximal single inflation time	0.65771	0.23273	2.82606	0.0047	Long inflation time
Unstable angina	0.57120	0.22765	2.50911	0.0127	Unstable angina
Stenosis before PTCA	0.40081	0.16932	2.36717	0.0179	High-grade stenosis

stenosis exceeded 2.5 mm (p = 0.001). Improvement of stenosis was also correlated with the recurrence rate. A stenosis reduction < 50% culminated in a restenosis rate of 35%, whereas a reduction > 70% was followed by a significantly lower restenosis rate of 24% (p = 0.042). A comparable trend with regard to absolute diameters did not reach statistical significance. The presence of intimal dissection after PTCA was associated with only a slightly lower rate of restenosis (24% vs 30%, ns).

Procedural variables

A maximal inflation pressure < 7 atm was followed by a significantly higher restenosis rate (32% vs 21%) as higher inflation pressures (p = 0.028, Table 2). The recurrence rate of lesions varied from 25% if the maximal single inflation time did not exceed 30 s, to 29% in patients with an inflation time of 30–60 s, and up to 45% if the maximal single inflation time was prolonged to > 60 s (p = 0.017). Duration of the total inflation time, which adds from all single inflation times, was also related to the restenosis rate. We found a restenosis rate of 27% in patients with a total inflation time < 120 s, 26% in patients with an inflation time of 120–240 s, but 37% if an inflation time > 240 s was used (p = 0.55).

A higher number of inflations and a high ratio of vessel/balloon diameter were also combined with a higher restenosis rate, without reaching statistical significance.

Multivariate analysis

A stepwise logistic regression procedure selected four variables independently related to a higher risk of restenosis (Table 3). These were in order of significance: 1) large residual stenosis (p = 0.0001), 2) long single inflation time (p = 0.0047), 3) unstable angina (p = 0.0127), and 4) high-grade stenosis before PTCA (p = 0.0179).

Discussion

Restenosis after successful PTCA remains a major challenge of this procedure. In large-scale series, restenosis rates were constantly found to be in a range of 30% [12, 15, 26], which compares also with the 29% restenosis rate in our study.

Univariate analysis of risk factors

Univariate analysis revealed two clinical factors to have a major influence on lesion recurrence, namely unstable angina and a short duration of symptoms preceding PTCA.

Both variables had been identified as risk factors for restenosis by previous large-scale studies [9, 12, 15, 22, 26]. The finding suggests that restenosis is more likely in younger active lesions.

Looking at pre-PTCA angiographic variables only the severity of the lesion was significantly correlated with an increased risk of subsequent restenosis. This finding is also in agreement with previous studies [12, 22]. Whereas Leimgruber [12] reported the site of lesions as being of major importance in predicting recurrence, we could not confirm this finding in our study. Leimgruber concluded that his result might be related to the use of relatively undersized balloons (3.0 mm) in coronary arteries with a wide luminal diameter and thus would reflect an insufficient dilatation rather than an inherent risk that the coronary artery itself undergoes lesion recurrence. The higher restenosis rate of proximal lesions in our patients may also be explained on this basis. A lower degree of improvement in luminal diameter narrowing was also correlated with a higher incidence of recurrent lesions, thus clarifying that elastic recoil does not have a major effect on lesion recurrence.

The post-PTCA result proved to be the most powerful predictor of restenosis. Accordingly, previous authors [5, 9, 10, 15, 26] also found a significantly higher restenosis rate in patients with a residual stenosis > 30%. Therefore, any effort during PTCA should be aimed to get a sufficient primary result. But this parameter should be subject to some criticism, as a noteworthy residual stenosis comes out to be a restenosis by itself. Furthermore, definition of restenosis in our group was directly influenced by this parameter.

The favorable influence of an uncomplicated dissection was reported by other authors [11, 15] and a similar tendency was observed in our patients. However, since intimal dissection increases the risk of major complications during PTCA the procedure should not be aimed to achieve intimal dissection.

Only little data is so far available on the influence of procedural factors on restenosis. An inflation pressure of > 7 atm was associated with a significantly lower restenosis rate in our patients group, whereas in accordance with Levine et al. [17] Leimgruber et al. did not find a favorable effect of higher inflation pressures and other authors even reported on adverse effects of high balloon pressures [20, 21, 29]. Considering that balloon pressure was not selected as an independent risk factor by multivariate analysis, the higher restenosis rate in our low-pressure group could merely be due to an insufficient primary result. Of course, well-controlled studies have to be done to further clarify these opposite findings. In contrast to a previous report [14] which suggested that prolonged application of balloon extension may improve primary and long-term results of angioplasty, we found a significantly higher restenosis rate if the maximal single or total inflation time was prolonged. Long inflation times have mainly been used in the very first patients of this series to get some information on ischemic tolerance during PTCA. Possibly, the unfavorable effect of prolonged inflation times may only be due to presumably better collaterals in this subgroup. Nevertheless, this data does not provide evidence that prolonged inflations might reduce the rate of lesion recurrence.

A higher number of inflations was also combined with an increase in recurrence rate without reaching a significant level. A study from the Montreal Heart Institute [9] and another report [3] revealed a significant relation of a higher restenosis rate to repeated balloon inflations. In a randomized trial, Uebis et al. [27] were the first to demonstrate that additional inflations in patients with a good initial result after one inflation were followed by a significantly higher lesion recurrence. Of course, a higher number of inflations may be needed to get a sufficient initial result and thus may only reflect the rigidity of the lesion. But in this case a higher risk of restenosis has to be considered. Accordingly, Uebis found the best long-term results in patients who showed a good angiographic result after one inflation only. A large ratio of balloon/vessel diameter has been proposed by other groups [6, 19, 28] to reduce the rate of lesion recurrence and a comparable tendency was seen in our patients. However, a recent randomized study [19] could demonstrate that a larger

Table 4. Multivariate analysis: risk factors for restenosis after PTCA.

	NHLBI 1984 n = 439	Atlanta 1986 n = 787	Present study 1989 n = 458
Male sex	+	0	0
History of MI	+	0	0
Bypass-Graft	+	−	−
Angina symptoms (CCS)	+	0	0
Intimal dissection	0	+	0
Final gradient	−°	+	−
Diseased vessel	0	+	0
Stenosis before PTCA	0	+*	+
Stenosis after PTCA	0	+	+
Unstable angina	0	+	+
Maximal single inflation time	−	−	+

+ significant
0 not significant
− not evaluated
° only included in univariate analysis
* total or subtotal occlusion (≥ 95% diameter stenosis) included

balloon/vessel ratio was combined with a significantly higher rate of acute complications. Therefore, selection of relatively oversized balloons should be avoided.

Multivariate analysis of risk factors

Multivariate analysis revealed four factors independently related to a higher risk of restenosis after PTCA (Table 4): 1) severity of stenosis before PTCA, 2) residual stenosis after PTCA, 3) presence of unstable angina, and 4) long inflation time. The first three variables had also been identified by Leimgruber et al. (Table 4). Data on maximal single inflation time had not been included in the NHLBI-report [12] nor in the Emory-report [15].

In addition, three other variables were found to be related to a higher risk of lesion recurrence in the Emory-report: presence of intimal dissection, final gradient > 15, and PTCA of the LAD.

Although there was a favorable trend for a lower restenosis rate in the presence of intimal dissection, this variable failed to reach statistical significance in our group. The final gradient was not routinely measured in our patients because of the inherent drawbacks of this method. Since there is a good correlation between translesional gradient and residual stenosis [1], these parameters may not be truly independent and thus only one of these variables should be included in multivariate analysis. The higher restenosis rate after PTCA of the LAD had not been confirmed by the NHLBI-report, nor in our patient group. This finding may be explained by a systematic bias, as Leimgruber himself concluded. None of the factors that had been found by multivariate analysis in the NHLBI-report could be confirmed by Leimgruber's report or in our study. Thus three variables have been identified by multivariate analysis in two independent large-scale studies: 1) severity of lesion before PTCA and 2) after PTCA, and 3) unstable angina.

Restenosis remains the most important limitation with regard to the long-term benefit of PTCA. Trials on various drug regimes after PTCA so far have yielded disappointing results [2, 30, 31]. Thus, there is still the challenge of defining any factor whose modification could reduce the problem. Since clinical and pre-PTCA variables cannot be modified, one should at least aim to achieve a good primary result. The important influence of the post-PTCA result on restenosis rate is documented by this and previous studies. Modification of the PTCA procedure with respect to short inflation time, higher inflation pressure, and avoidance of unnecessary repeated inflations, as long as the primary result is sufficient, may be of benefit in reducing the risk of restenosis after successful PTCA. Therefore, the role of procedural factors should be further evaluated in randomized studies.

Conclusion

To identify risk factors for restenosis we evaluated data in 473 patients with single-vessel PTCA and control angiography after 6 months.

Restenosis, defined as 1) loss > 50% of the initial gain and 2) stenosis > 50% was found in 138 patients (29.2%). Univariate analysis revealed eight factors related to restenosis: 1) Duration of symptoms < 1 month (p = 0.005), 2) unstable angina (p = 0.004), 3) high grade stenosis before PTCA (p = 0.014), 4) large residual stenosis after PTCA (p = 0.001), 5) insufficient improvement of stenosis (p = 0.042), 6) prolonged single inflation time (p = 0.017), 7) prolonged total inflation time (p = 0.055), and 8) low inflation pressure (p = 0.028).

Multivariate analysis revealed four factors significantly related to restenosis: 1) large residual stenosis after PTCA (p = 0.0001), 2) prolonged single inflation time (p = 0.0047), 3) unstable angina (p = 0.0127), and 4) high grade stenosis before PTCA (p = 0.0179).

Modification of procedural factors might be helpful to reduce the risk of restenosis after successful PTCA.

References

1. Anderson HV, Roubin GS, Leimgruber PP, Cox WR, Douglas JS Jr, King SB III, Grüntzing AR (1986) Measurement of trans-stenotic pressure gradient during percutaneous transluminal coronary angioplasty. Circulation 73: 1223–1230
2. Corcos T, David PR, Val PG, Renkin J, Dangoisse V, Rapold HG, Bourassa MG (1985) Failure of diltiazem to prevent restenosis after percutaneous transluminal coronary angioplasty. Am Heart J 109: 926–931
3. Dangoisse V, Guiteras Val P, David PR, Lesperance J, Crepeau J, Dydra I, Bourassa MG (1982) Recurrence of stenosis after successful percutaneous transluminal coronary angioplasty (PTCA). Circulation 66: II–331
4. David PR, Renkin J, Moise A, Dangoisse V, Guiteras PG, Bourassa MG (1984) Can patient selection and optimization of technique reduce the rate of restenosis after percutaneous transluminal coronary angioplasty? J Am Coll Cardiol 3: 470 (abst)
5. DiSciascio G, Cowley MJ, Vetrovec GW (1986) Angiographic patterns of restenosis after angioplasty of multiple coronary arteries. Am J Cardiol 58: 922–925
6. Duprat G, David PR, Lesperance J, Val PG, Fines P, Robert P, Bourassa MG (1984) An optimal size of balloon catheter is critical to angiographic success early after PTCA. Circulation 70: II–295
7. Grüntzig AR (1978) Transluminal dilatation of coronary-artery stenosis (letter to the editor). Lancet 1: 263
8. Grüntzig AR, Senning A, Siegenthaler, WE (1979) Nonoperative dilatation of coronary-artery stenosis: percutaneous transluminal coronary angioplasty. N Engl J Med 301: 61–68
9. Guiteras Val PG, Bourassa MG, Davis PR, Bonan R, Crépeau J, Dyrda I, Lespérance J (1987) Restenosis after successful percutaneous transluminal coronary angioplasty: the Montreal Heart Institute Experience. Am J Cardiol 60: 50B–55B
10. Hoffmeister JM, Whitworth HB, Leimgruber PP, Abi-Mansour P, Tate JM, Grüntzig AR (1985) Analysis of anatomic and procedural factors related to restenosis after double lesion coronary angioplasty (PTCA). Circulation 72: II–398
11. Hollman J, Galan K, Franco I, Simpfendorfer C, Fatica K, Beck G (1986) Recurrent stenosis after coronary angioplasty. J Am Coll Cardiol 7: 20A

12. Holmes DR, Vliestra RE, Smith HC, Vetrovec GW, Kent KM, Cowley MJ, Faxon DP, Grüntzig AR, Kelsey SF, Detre KM, Van Raden MJ, Mock MB (1984) Restenosis after percutaneous transluminal coronary angioplasty (PTCA): a report from the PTCA Registry of the National Heart, Lung, and Blood Institute. Am J Cardiol 53: 77C

13. Kaltenbach M, Kober G, Scherer D, Vallbracht C (1985) Recurrence rate after successful coronary angioplasty. Eur Heart J 6: 276–281

14. Kaltenbach M, Kober G (1982) Can prolonged application of pressure improve the results of coronary angioplasty (PTCA)? Circulation 66: III–123 (abst)

15. Leimgruber PP, Roubin GS, Hollman J, Cotsonis GA, Meier B, Douglas JS, King III SP, Grüntzing AR (1986) Restenosis after sucessful coronary angioplasty in patients with single-vessel disease. Circulation 73: 710–717

16. Levine S, Ewels CJ, Rosing DR, Kent KM (1985) Coronary angioplasty: clinical and angiographic follow-up. Am J Cardiol 55: 673

17. Levine S, Ewels CJ, Rosing DR, Kent KM (1983) Restenosis (R) following transluminal coronary angioplasty (TCA). Circulation 68: III–96

18. Mabin TA, Holmes DR Jr, Smith HC, Vlietstra RE, Reeder GS, Breshnahan JF, Bove AA, Hammes LN, Elveback LR, Orszulak TA (1985) Follow-up clinical results in patients undergoing percutaneous transluminal coronary angioplasty. Circulation 71: 754–760

19. Mata LA, Bosch X, David PR, Rapold HJ, Corcos T, Bourassa MG (1985) Clinical and angiographic assessment 6 months after double vessel percutaneous coronary angioplasty. J Am Coll Cardiol 6: 1239–1244

20. Marantz T, Williams DO, Reinert S, Gewirtz H, Most AS (1984) Predictors of restenosis after successful coronary angioplasty. Circulation 70: II–176

21. Meier B, Grüntzig AR, King SB III, Douglas JS, Hollmann J, Ischinger T, Galan K (1984) Higher balloon dilatation pressure in coronary angioplasty. Am Heart J 107: 619–622

22. Meyer J, Schmitz HJ, Kiesslich T, Erbel R, Krebs W, Schulz W, Bardos P, Minale C, Messmer BJ, Effert S (1983) Percutaneous transluminal coronary angioplasty in patients with stable and unstable angina pectoria: Analysis of early and late results. Am Heart J 106: 973–980

23. Meyer J, Böcker B, Erbel R, Bardos P, Messmer BJ, Effert S (1980) Treatment of unstable angina with transluminal coronary angioplasty (PTCA). Circulation 62: 160

24. Meyer J, Schmitz H, Erbel R, Kiesslich T, Böcker-Josephs B, Krebs W, Braun PC, Bardos P, Minale C, Messmer BJ, Effert S (1981) Treatment of unstable angina pectoris with percutaneous transluminal coronary angioplasty. Cathet Cardiovasc Diagn 7: 361–371

25. Myler RK, Topol EJ, Shaw RE, Stertzer SH, Clark DA, Fishman-Rosen J, Murphy MC (1987) Multiple vessel coronary angioplasty: Classification, results and patterns of restenosis in 494 consecutive patients. Cathet Cardiovasc Diagn 13: 1–15

26. Rapold HJ, David PR, Guiteras Val P, Mata AL, Crean PA, Bourassa MG (1987) Restenosis and its determinants in first and repeat coronary angioplasty. Eur Heart J 8: 575–586

27. Schmitz E, v Dahl J, Uebis R, Blome R, v Essen R, Hanrath P (1989) Rezidivrate nach erfolgreicher PTCA: Keine Reduktion durch eine Mehrfachinsufflation des Ballons. Z Kardiol 78: I–56 (abst)

28. Schmitz HJ, v Essen R, Meyer J, Effert S (1984) The role of balloon size for acute and late angiographic results in coronary angioplasty. Circulation 70: II–295

29. Shaw RE, Myler RK, Fishman-Rosen J, Murphy MC, Stertzer SH, Topol EJ (1986) Clinical and morphologic factors in prediction of restenosis after multiple vessel angiography. J Am Coll Cardiol 7: 63A

30. Thornton MA, Grüntzig AR, Hollman J, King SB, Douglas JS (1984) Coumadin and aspirin in prevention of recurrence after transluminal coronary angioplasty: a randomized study. Circulation 69: 721–727

31. Whitworth HB, Roubin GS, Hollman J, Meier B, Leimgruber PP, Douglas JS, King SB III, Grüntzig AR (1986) Effect of nifedipine on recurrent stenosis after percutaneous transluminal coronary angioplasty. J Am Coll Cardiol 8: 1271–1276

Author's address:
Hans J. Rupprecht, M.D.
II. Medizinische Klinik
Johannes-Gutenberg-Universität
Langenbeckstr. 1
6500 Mainz, FRG

Restenosis after Perfusion Balloon Catheter Use: Initial Experience

J. Krülls-Münch, E. Frantz, U. Sauer, H. Oswald, E. Fleck

German Heart Institute, Berlin, FRG

Introduction

PTCA is a widely recognized safe method to treat coronary artery disease (CAD) and is used in addition to medical therapy and bypass surgery. One of its major accompanying problems is the rate of restenosis [1]. Recent studies have shown the benefit of prolongation of balloon inflation time [2]. The occurrence of myocardial ischemia during conventional PTCA is the limiting factor for inflation time, especially in the case of left main coronary artery (LMCA) stenosis and lesions close to the aortal ostium. There are some recommendations concerning protection of myocardium during transient artery occlusion, e.g., administration of propanolol during inflation [3]. Another possible method is the use of autoperfusion balloon catheters that allow passive myocardial perfusion during balloon inflation through a central lumen and multiple side holes in the shaft proximal and distal to the balloon. (Fig. 1). In 1988, Stack and Quigley published the first experience with this intrument in humans [4]. They concluded that ischemic symptoms and signs during PTCA were significantly reduced.

The aim of our study was to investigate the rate of restenosis by prolongation of inflation time with autoperfusion balloon catheter.

Patients and methods

From May, 1988 to May, 1989, 28 patients (pts) (23 male/5 female, mean age 55.4 years) were investigated; they showed high grade stenoses of LMCA (in four pts), LAD (in 20 pts), LCX (in one pt) and RCA (in three pts). Seven patients had already undergone PTCA and showed restenosis. Seven patients had a prior myocardial infarction, and four patients had undergone previous bypass surgery. Angioplasty was performed by the Judkins femoral approach. Systemic anticoagulation was achieved with heparin i.v. 10 000 IU at the beginning of the procedure. Balloon inflation and vessel dilation was maintained until electrocardiographic or hemodynamic signs of ischemia were evident on otherwise up to

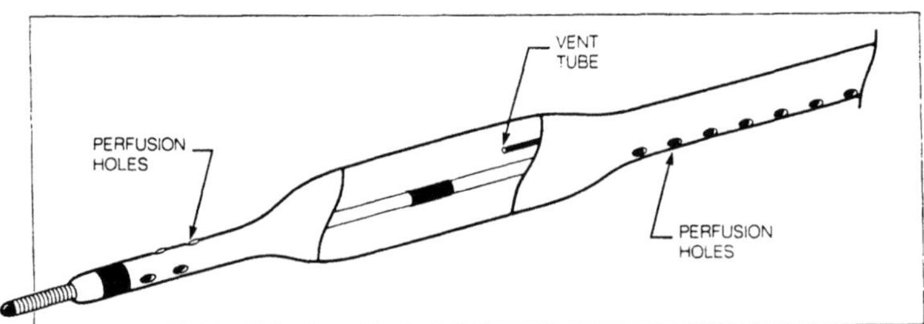

Fig. 1. Autoperfusion balloon catheter: passive coronary perfusion during balloon inflation is permitted by a central lumen that ends in perfusion holes proximal and distal to the balloon.

25 min. Ischemic events were defined as elevation or depression of ST-segments exceeding 3 mm in any ECG-lead or increase of mean pulmonary artery pressure (PAm) of more than 10 mmHg.

Results

Balloon inflation time and pressure, ischemic events

Twenty-six patients underwent an uncomplicated procedure, two patients had a circular dissection in the attacked vessel and required elective bypass surgery. Balloon inflation time was 665 s, ranging from 360 to 1500 s. Balloon inflation pressure ranged from 3.0 to

Table 1. Balloon inflation pressures and sizes.

Balloon pressure (atm)	No. of pts	Balloon size (F)	No. of pts
3.0	9	2.5	6
3.5	2	3.0	15
4.0	13	3.5	6
4.5	1	4.0	1
5.0	2		
6.0	1		

5.5 atm. Pressures and balloon sizes are shown in Table 1.Ischemic events as defined before were registered in 17/28 patients, as shown in Table 2.

Table 2. Incidence of ischemic events.

No. of Pts. with:	ST-segment unchanged	ST-segment elevation/depression
PAm unchanged	11	10
PAm-increase > 10 mmHG	2	5

Primary stenosis reduction

Results were evaluated by quantitative coronary angiography. The cross-sectional area of the attacked lesions was 0.82 ± 0.39 mm^2 before PTCA and 3.55 ± 1.88 mm^2 after PTCA. This led to an improvement of coronary flow reserve from 2.48 ± 0.76 before PTCA to 4.87 ± 0.19 after PTCA. The other primary results of PTCA are given in Table 3.

Table 3.. Primary results of PTCA.

Stenosis as % reduction of:	Area	Diameter
Before PTCA	92.4 ± 3.4	73.1 ± 5.9
After PTCA	49.6 ± 10.6	33.1 ± 10.7

Table 4.

Quantitative data of 22/28 pts:	With good results n = 12	With restenosis n = 10
Area (mm^2)	2.82 ± 1.31	1.68 ± 1.24
Area reduction (%)	35.2 ± 16.5	79.7 ± 14.7
Diameter reduct. (%)	20.7 ± 11.0	60.5 ± 22.9
Coron. flow reserve	4.98 ± 0.06	3.28 ± 1.91

Follow-up

Twenty-two of 28 patients were investigated 2 months after the primary PTCA. Ten patients showed restenosis (45%) and 12 patients showed good results. Two patients with LMCA stenosis and four patients with LAD-stenosis underwent a second successful PTCA, whereas four patients needed elective coronary bypass surgery. There was no difference between the two groups in basic data and balloon inflation time or pressure. Quantitative data of the target stenoses are given for both groups in Table 4.

Conclusions

The initial experience with autoperfusion balloon catheters shows no advantage considering restenosis, but with their use it is possible to dilate LMCA or near-ostial stenosis of coronary arteries without provocation of severe ischemia. Further investigations are needed to define the group of patients who can profit from this treatment method.

References

1. Blackshear JL, O'Callaghan WG, Califf RM. (1987) Medical approaches to prevention of restenosis after coronary angioplasty. J Am Coll Cardiol; 9:834–48
2. Kaltenbach M, Koberg G. (1982) Can prolonged application of pressure improve the results of coronary angioplasty? (PTCA) (abstract) Circulation; 66: (suppl II):II–123
3. Feldmann RL, Macdonald RG, Hill JA, Limacher MC, Conti CR, Pepine CJ. (1986) Effect of Propanolol on myocardial ischemia during acute coronary occlusion. Circulation 73, No. 4, 727–733
4. Stack RS, Quigley PJ, Collins G, Phillips HR. (1988) Perfusion balloon catheter. Am J Cardiol; 61, 77–80
5. Quigley PJ, Hinohara T, Phillips HR, Peter RH, Behar VS, Kong Y, Sionton, CA, Perez JA, Stack RS. (1988) Myocardial Protection during coronary angioplasty with an autoperfusion balloon catheter in humans. Circulation; 78:1128–1134
6. Turi ZG, Campbell CA, Gottimukkala MV, Kloner RA. (1987) Preservation of distal coronary perfusion during prolonged balloon inflation with an autoperfusion angioplasty catheter. Circulation. 75, No. 6, 1273–1280

Author's address:
Klinik für Innere Medizin – Kardiologie
Deutsches Herzzentrum Berlin
Augustenburger Platz 1
1000 Berlin 65, FRG

Pathologist's View on Restenosis

C. Düber

Institut für Klinische Strahlenkunde, Universitätskliniken, Mainz, FRG

Restenosis after PTCA is a pathological process related to the healing mechanism following balloon-induced arterial wall injury.

In 1963, a year before Dotter reported on "transluminal treatment of arteriosclerotic obstruction" [6] "a new method for the production of thrombi by overdilatation of the vessel wall" was introduced by Baumgartner [2, 3]. In these papers the pathological changes after dilatation including neointimal proliferation were described without knowledge that this process might become important in restenosis after angioplasty. The first autopsy study on restenosis after therapeutic dilatation appeared 20 years later by Essed et al. [8].

The following description of the healing process and restenosis after PTCA is based on own observations in six patients who died 8 to 52 days after angioplasty [7], and a review of the literature reporting on autopsy material [1, 5, 9, 11–19].

Platelet aggregation

In the acute phase after PTCA, when injury to the intima and media has occurred, small platelet thrombi can be observed on the denuded original or the newly created intimal surface. Platelet aggregation is paralleled by thin fibrin deposits on the luminal surface.

In this early phase after PTCA there are complex (incompletely understood) biochemical interactions between platelets, mural thrombi, cells from the circulating blood, intimal and medial cells [4, 10]. One of the results of these interactions is a neointimal proliferation of smooth muscle cells.

Neointimal proliferation

A few days after PTCA a thin interrupted layer or small aggregates of smooth muscle cells can be observed on the rough intimal surface or the luminal surface of subintimal or submedial dissection clefts leading to smoothening of the neolumen (Fig. 1).

In patients with restenosis an extensive neointimal proliferation with considerable reobstruction has been noted in several autopsy cases including one patient from our own study who died 52 days after PTCA. In this patient the whole luminal surface of the dilated artery consisting of the original intimal plaque, a mural thrombus, the torn ends of the intimal and medial flaps, and the media (outer aspect) and adventitia (inner aspect) in the region of submedial dissection was coated by a thick layer of neointima (Fig. 2).

The neointima consisted of smooth muscle cells within a loose intercellular matrix and it was clearly differentiated from preexisting intimal plaque material. In summary the healing process after PTCA includes platelet aggregation and thrombus formation in the early phase and neointimal proliferation of smooth muscle cells in the later phase.

It is not known from pathological studies why neointima formation results in small coverage of the neolumen in most patients, and restenosis by extensive proliferation in others.

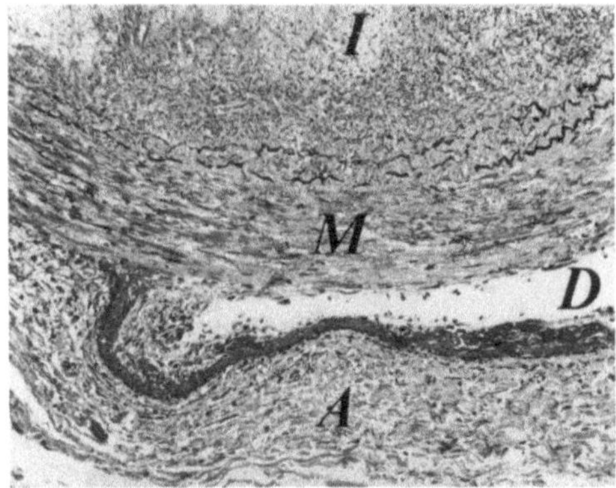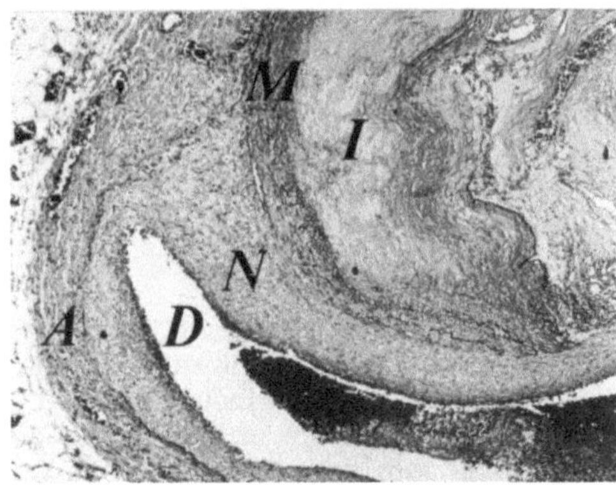

Fig. 1. Coronary artery 8 days after PTCA: submedial dissection cleft (D) covered with fibrin deposits and small aggregates of smooth muscle cells. I = intima; M = media; A = adventitia.

Fig. 2. Coronary artery 52 days after PTCA: submedial dissection cleft (D) filled with recent thrombus and covered with thick layer of neointimal proliferation of smooth muscle cells (N). I = intima; M = media; A = adventitia.

References

1. Austin GE, Ratliff NB, Hollman J, Phillips DF (1985) Intimal proliferation of smooth muscle cells as an explanation for recurrent coronary artery stenosis after percutaneous transluminal coronary angioplasty. J Am Coll Cardiol 6: 369–375
2. Baumgartner HR (1963) Eine neue Methode zur Erzeugung von Thromben durch gezielte Überdehnung der Gefäßwand. Z ges exp Med 137: 227–247
3. Baumgartner HR, Studer A (1963) Gezielte Überdehnung der Aorta abdominalis am normo-und hypercholesterinämischen Kaninchen. Path Mikrobiol 26: 129–148
4. Chesebro JH, Lam JYT, Badimon L, Fuster V (1987) Restenosis after arterial angioplasty: a hemorheologic response to injury. Am J Cardiol 60: 10B–16B
5. Colavita PG, Ideker RE, Reimer KA, Hackel DB, Stack RS (1986) The spectrum of pathology associated with percutaneous transluminal coronary angioplasty during acute myocardial infarction. J Am Coll Cardiol 8: 855–860
6. Dotter CT, Judkins MP (1964) Transluminal treatment of arteriosclerotic obstruction. Description of a new technique and a preliminary report of its application. Circulation 30: 654–670
7. Düber C, Jungbluth A, Rumpelt HJ, Erbel R, Meyer J, Thoenes W (1986) Morphology of the coronary arteries after combined thrombolysis and percutaneous transluminal angioplasty for acute myocardial infarction. Am J Cardiol 58, 698–703
8. Essed CE, Van den Brand M, Becker AE (1983) Transluminal coronary angioplasty and early restenosis. Fibrocellular occlusion after wall laceration. Br Heart J 49: 393–396
9. Giraldo AA, Esposo OM, Meis JM (1985) Intimal hyperplasia as a cause of restenosis after percutaneous transluminal coronary angioplasty. Arch Pathol Lab Med 109: 173–175
10. Gravanis MB (1988) The enigma of restenosis after percutaneous transluminal coronary angioplasty. Am J Cardiovasc Pathol 2: 1–5
11. Kohchi K, Takebayashi S, Block PC, Hiroki T, Nobuyoshi M (1987) Arterial changes after percutaneous transluminal coronary angioplasty. Am J Coll Cardiol 10: 592–599
12. Mittal V, Karl EM, Atkinson JB, Virmani R (1986) Early and late morphologic changes after transluminal balloon angioplasty of the iliac arteries. Am J Cardiol 58: 182–184
13. Saber RS, Edwards WD, Holmes DR, Vlietstra RE, Reeder GS (1988) Balloon angioplasty of aortocoronary saphenous vein bypass grafts: a histopathologic study of six grafts from five patients with emphasis on restenosis and embolic complications. J Am Coll Cardiol 12: 1501–1509
14. Schneider J, Grüntzig A (1985) Percutaneous transluminal angioplasty. Morphological findings in 3 patients. Path Res Prac 180: 348–352
15. Ueda M, Becker AE, Fujimoto T (1987) Pathological changes induced by repeated percutaneous transluminal coronary angioplasty. Br Heart J 58: 635–643

16. Waller BF, Gorfinkel HJ, Rogers FJ, Kent KM, Roberts WC (1984) Early and late morphological changes in major epicardial coronary arteries after percutaneous transluminal coronary angioplasty. Am J Cardiol 53: 42C–47C
17. Waller BF, Rothbaum DA, Pinkerton CA, Cowley MJ, Linnemeier TJ, Orr C, Irons M, Helmuth RA, Wills ER, Aust C (1987) Status of the myocardium and infarct-related coronary artery in 19 necropsy patients with acute recanalization using pharmacologic (streptokinase, r-tissue plasminogen activator), mechanical (percutaneous transluminal coronary angioplasty) or combined types of reperfusion therapy. J Am Coll Cardiol 9: 785–801
18. Waller BC, Pinkerton CA, Foster LN (1987) Morphologic evidence of accelerated left main coronary artery stenosis: a late complication of percutaneous transluminal balloon angioplasty of the proximal left anterior descending coronary artery. J Am Coll Cardiol 9: 1019–1023
19. Zarins CK, Lu C, Gewertz BL, Lyon RT, Rush DS, Glagov S (1982) Arterial disruption and remodelling following balloon dilatation. Surgery 92: 1086–1095

Author's address:
Dr C. Düber
Institut für Klinische Strahlenkunde
Universitätskliniken
Langenbeckstraße 1
6500 Mainz, FRG

Final Remarks

Prevention of Complications by Angioplasters' Training and Patient Selection

G. O. Hartzler

Kansas City, Missouri, USA

Introduction

The volume was designed to present expert opinions on invasive cardiologic treatment, especially PTCA, concentrating upon complications of angioplasty techniques. Like many other invasive forms of cardiologic and medical treatment certain harms and pitfalls of these treatment strategies can be prevented by accumulting experience about the treatment techniques.

In contrast to many treatment forms, we are provided with exact data on incidence and preconditions for unsuccessful outcome and complications of coronary angioplasty, starting from the first clinical uses in 1977 and 1978. On the basis of these data, we are able to give certain recommendations for training of those who perform angioplasty and selection of patients, both of which have proven to be important for the prevention of complications [1, 6].

The learning curve of PTCA: Increasing rate of successful procedures

The deliberate registry of data of PTCA-patients, performed by the NHLBI 1977–1981 (n = 3.079) and again in 1985–6 (n = 2.094), showed a markedly increasing rate of successful procedures from the beginning to the later years of performing angioplasty [2, 3]. With these data a so-called PTCA "learning curve" could be constructed [5]. Annual success rates are given in the first figure, showing the "learning curve" from June 1980 to June 1987, for 5 operators at the Mid-America Heart Institute in Kansas City.

The second figure shows individual learning curves for the 5 operators related to case-volume experience.

There is not only a learning curve for the overall success-rate of PTCA, collecting all data from different centers, but also a personal learning curve for each angioplaster. The NHLBI-data showed a clear interrelation between the number of procedures that was performed at a certain site, and the angiographically defined success-rate. This was reflected by a simultaneous decline in the necessity for elective coronary surgery as primary failure decreased [4].

During the same period, rates for emergency CABG and myocardial infarction decreased modestly with investigator experience. The data are given in the following table.

Table 1. Success rate and bad outcome in the first 150 cases of PTCA.

	Number of cases		
	< 50	50–149	> 150
Success-rate	55.1%	65.6%	76.7%
Elective CABG	24.4%	15.7%	10.8%
Emergency CABG	8.5%	5.2%	5.0%
In-hospital-MI	7.5%	4.3%	5.4%

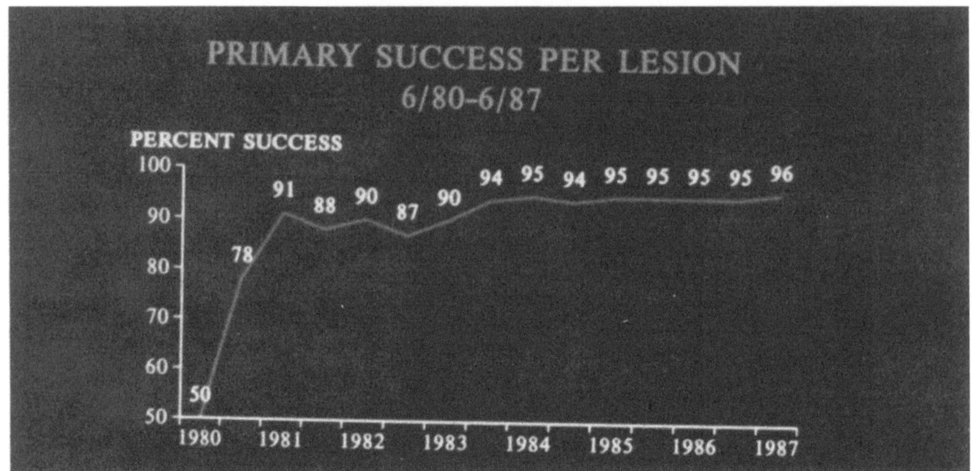

Fig. 1. "PTCA learning curve" (primary success per lesion attacked) for 5 operators at the Mid-America Heart Institute in Kansas City from June 1980 to June 1987.

As has been noted by B. Meier and A. Gruentzig [5], the initial steep upslope of the learning curve is mainly caused by growing skill of the particular operator, whereas the flatter part seems to be secondary to improvements in technical equipment.

An interesting aspect is the nearly unchanged rate of complications; perhaps the reason is that two factors are competitive: as experience increases, fewer emergency situations will occur, but simultaneously, more "high-risk" patients will be accepted for the procedure.

Training of angioplaster

The PTCA "learning curve" today largely reflects the effect of operator experience on procedural outcome.

The performance of PTCA is not equivalent to the performance of coronary angiography. Differences exist in the requirement of greater manipulative skills and for more complex judgements during the procedure. Increased procedural risks (morbidity/mortality 20 times as high) create greater stresses for the operator.

Operator experience includes:
– technical skills;
– adequate judgement for patient selection and management strategies;
– knowledge of and familiarity with devices;
– ability to manage complications;
– judgement of his own abilities.

Ideally, the PTCA operator should have passed intensive training before performing the first procedure. Today, the standards for comparing procedural outcomes are contemporary experiences rather than the historic data reported above. To reach this standard, the following experiences are suggested for optimal training:
– 500–1,000 unsupervised coronary angiograms during post-fellowship;
– institutional and peer recognition for competence;
– completion of training courses;
– in-laboratory observation;
– assistance to experienced operator for 25–30 cases.

Ideally, for the first cases, the following conditions should be met:
– assistance by experienced operator for 25–30 cases;

152

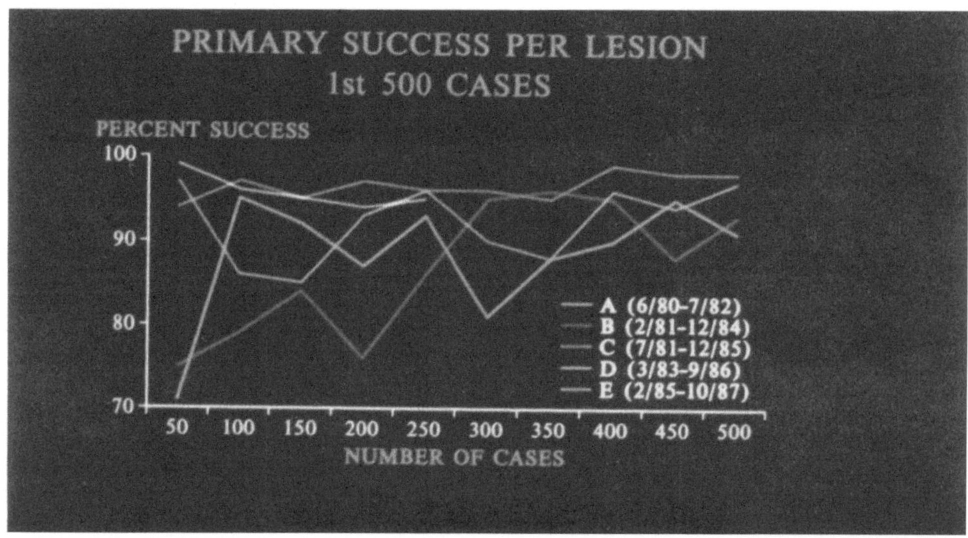

Fig. 2. Individual learning curves (primary success per lesion attacked) for 5 operators related to case volume experience.

– deliberate and restrictive patient selection for the first 100 cases;
– immediate availability of experienced operator;
– review of complications with experienced operator.
   Sufficient training success can be verified if the following optimal results are gained during the first 100 cases of PTCA:
– primary success 90%;
– emergency CABG < 5%;
– mortality ≤ 1%.
   An angioplaster may be defined as "beginning" during the first 100 cases, "intermediate" during case 100–500, and "advanced" after having performed 500 angioplasties.

Patient selection

Patient selection needs to be adequate to these different levels of training. In the following, indications and contraindications are listed for each level of operator experience.

Beginning operator

Current indications, including:
– documented myocardial ischemia;
– normal or mildly depressed left ventricular function (EF > 45%);
– single-vessel and single-lesion disease;
– subtotal stenosis length < 20 mm.

Intermediate operator

Indications	Relative Contraindications
– multivessel disease	– left main coronary artery disease
– complete occlusions	– LMCA-equivalent disease
– multilesion dilatation	– only remaining coronary vessel
– acute infarction intervention	– extremely poor LV function
	– elderly patients (with multilesion dilatation)

Advanced operator

Indications	Relative Contraindications
– "protected" LMCA disease	– "unprotected" LMCA disease
– LMCA-equivalent disease	– multiple restenosis
– only remaining coronary vessel	– selected patients who can be more
– poor LV function	completely revascularized with

– elderly patients (with multi-
    lesion dilatation +/− poor LV-
        function)
	bypass surgery than would be possible
	with PTCA

Conclusions

Training in PTCA is a continuous process with results largely influenced by operator experience.

Cautious, deliberate, and controlled acquisition of experience is required to achieve high primary success, low morbidity and mortality, and for applying PTCA to complex patient subsets.

References

1. ACC/AHA Task Force on Assessment of Diagnostic and Therapeutic Cardiovascular Procedures (Subcommittee on Percutaneous Transluminal Coronary Angioplasty) (1988) Guidelines for Percutaneous Transluminal Coronary Angioplasty. J Am Coll Cardiol 12 529–45.
2. Dorros G, Cowley MJ, Janke L, Kelsey SF, Mullin SM, Van Raden M (1984) In-Hospitality Mortality Rate in the National Heart, Lung, and Blood Institute Percutaneous Transluminal Coronary Angioplasty Registry. Am J Cardiol 53 Suppl. C 17C–21C.
3. Holmes DR, Holubkov R, Vlietstra RE, Kelsey SF, Reeder GS, Dorros G, Williams DO, Cowley MJ, Faxon DP, Kent KM, Bentivoglio LG, Detre K (1988) Comparison of Complications During Percutaneous Transluminal Coronary Angioplasty from 1977 to 1981 and from 1985 to 1986: The National Heart, Lung, and Blood Institute Percutaneous Transluminal Coronary Angioplasty Registry. J Am Coll Cardiol 12:1149–55.
4. Kelsey SF, Mullin SM, Detre KM, Mitchell H, Cowley MJ, Gruentzig AR, Kent KM (1984) Effect of Investigator Experience on Percutaneous Transluminal Coronary Angioplasty. Am J Cardiol 53 Suppl. C: 56C–64C.
5. Meier B, Gruentzig AR (1984) Learning Curve for Percutaneous Transluminal Coronary Angioplasty: Skill, Technology or Patient Selection. Am J Cardiol 53 Suppl. C: 65C–66C.
6. Williams DO, Gruentzig A, Kent KM, Myler RK, Stertzer SH, Bentivoglio L, Bourassa M, Block P, Cowley M, Detre K, Dorros G, Gosselin A, Simpson J, Passamani E, Mullin S (1982) Guidelines for the Performance of Percutaneous Transluminal Coronary Angioplasty. Circulation 66:693–4.

Author's address;
Geoffrey O. Hartzier M.D., Medical Plaza II-20, 4320 Wornall Road, Kansas City, MO. 64111, USA

This publication was made possible by a generous grant from:

Advanced Cardiovascular Systems, Inc.

3200 Lakeside Drive
Santa Clara, California, 95054, USA

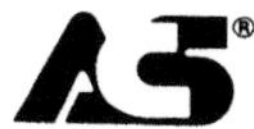